TREAT YOUR OWN STRAINS, SPRAINS AND BRUISES

By:

Robert Lindsay, *Dip. Phty (Otago), ADP (OMT), Dip. MT*
Grant Watson, *Dip. Phys. (Auckland), ADP (OMT), Dip. MT, Dip. MDT*
Donna Hickmott, *Dip. Phys. (Auckland), ADP (OMT), Dip. MT*
Lillian Bruynel, *Dip. Phys. (Auckland), ADP (OMT), Dip. MT*
Ann Broadfoot, *Dip. Phty (Otago), ADP (OMT), Dip. MT*

Edited by:
Paula Van Wijmen, *Dip. Phty (Neth), Dip. MT, Dip. MDT*

SPINAL PUBLICATIONS (N.Z.) LTD
1994

*This book is dedicated to all
our families and friends who
gave their continual support
to this project*

ISBN 0-9598049-4-3

PANIC PAGE

If you have just injured yourself:

FIRST-AID
for
strains, sprains and bruises
The RICE method of Self-Treatment

Rest	Stop immediately what you are doing.
Ice	Apply an ice or cold pack to the injury site for up to fifteen minutes. Warning: To prevent an ice burn place a damp towel between skin and ice pack.
Compression	Remove the ice or cold pack and apply a firm bandage.
Elevation	Elevate the injured limb in a supported position above the level of your heart.

DO NOT:

—apply heat

—massage your injury

—drink alcohol

**as these activities increase
bleeding and swelling**

**Now that you have successfully completed the first stage
of self-treatment, read on!**

ABOUT THE AUTHORS

The authors are New Zealand physiotherapists with postgraduate qualifications in manipulative therapy. They firmly believe in the important role of education and self-treatment within the scope of physiotherapy. They maintain that, given the essential information, people generally are able to successfully treat and prevent recurrence of many of the strains, sprains and bruises that frequently occur in daily life.

Physiotherapists with a postgraduate qualification in manipulative therapy specialise in the treatment of disturbances in the musculo-skeletal system. In the U.S.A. such therapists are known as orthopaedic physical therapists.

SPECIAL ACKNOWLEDGEMENT

We sincerely thank Paula Van Wijmen, Dip. Phty (Neth), Dip. MT, Dip. MDT, for editing our manuscript. Her dedicated contribution to clarifying and expanding our concepts has helped to ensure the material presented in this book is both precise in content and readily accessible to the reader.

As a manipulative physiotherapist Paula is involved with the treatment and rehabilitation of acute and chronic sports injuries as well as spinal and general musculo-skeletal problems at the Te Aro Physiotherapy clinic in Wellington, New Zealand.

ACKNOWLEDGEMENTS

We are indebted to Robin McKenzie, OBE, FCSP, FNZSP (Hon), Dip. MT, for his generous support and encouragement that has made the production of this book possible. Robin is a New Zealand physiotherapist who is internationally recognised for his pioneering work in the field of self-treatment for back and neck pain.

Our special thanks go to Dr Ruth Highet, MB ChB, Dip. Obs., Dip. Sports Med. (London), FACSP, FACSM, for reviewing our book. Her in-depth knowledge of medical and musculo-skeletal disorders affecting men, women and children has been a valued contribution to the production of this book.

Our thanks also go to Susan Battye, MA (Loughborough), Dip. Drama in Education, Dip. Teaching, for editing the manuscript in its final stages from a non-medical person's perspective; photographer Kerry Doherty, Doherty's Studio, Thames; models for the photographs Jackie Piper, Dip. Phty (Otago), Dip. MT, Auckland, and Bernie Bourke, Thames; illustrator Barbara Pine, Auckland; proofreader and typist Julieann Pound; and typists Susan Maxwell, Kelly Marshall, Jan Richards and Sonja Williams; proofreader Eric Toplis, Thames.

FOREWORD

It gives me great pleasure to contribute this foreword to *Treat Your Own Strains, Sprains and Bruises*. Judging by the popularity of my own books *Treat Your Own Back and Treat Your Own Neck*, it would appear that the sufferer of injury will avidly practise procedures of self-help, if those procedures can be shown to relieve his or her pain and accelerate the recovery of normal day to day function. If the recommended procedures also help reduce progressive injury and prevent recurrence, so much the better.

It is time for us to recognise that, following injury, all life has a remarkable capacity to repair itself and recover. Nature has equipped us with a self-repairing mechanism that requires little assistance to work efficiently. Too often we rush needlessly to our doctor or physiotherapist for assistance when all that is required is the right mixture of rest and exercise. It is now well-recognised that the nutrition of our joints and their associated structures will be impaired if movement is inadequate. Providing we rest for the appropriate length of time and then commence movement in the appropriate manner, recovery will certainly follow.

The authors of *Treat Your Own Strains, Sprains and Bruises* have pooled their combined experiences to produce a carefully and skilfully written book. The information to follow will assist all of us who experience the common problems that occur in our day to day living on the planet Earth. The authors have been careful to restrict their advice to the treatment of uncomplicated soft tissue injuries. Nevertheless, the information within will be of benefit to prevent or reduce the consequences of long-term impairment of function that so often appears in later life.

This book describes how you may treat your own strains, sprains and bruises. By carefully following the advice within, you should recover rapidly and completely from the common injuries arising from modern daily living.

Robin McKenzie, OBE, FCSP, FNZSP (Hon), Dip.MT

FOREWORD

With the increased awareness of the benefits of regular exercise and improved physical fitness on our health and well-being, we are seeing a larger number of people experiencing musculo-skeletal injuries. There is also an increase in patients presenting with chronic injuries and disability arising from incomplete rehabilitation of a previously injured part. Incomplete rehabilitation causes muscle weakness, loss of balance and sometimes early joint damage and arthritis. Often this could have been prevented by early and complete treatment and full rehabilitation of the injury.

As in all areas of health and medicine, more than ever before, patients want to know in plain language what the likely diagnosis is, what they should and should not do to hasten their recovery, and when they can return to their chosen exercise, sport, job or other activity involving the musculo-skeletal system.

This book provides sensible advice for the immediate and ongoing treatment of minor musculo-skeletal injuries in adults as well as for a return to activity after injury. It also indicates when people might require advice from a doctor or physiotherapist to rule out problems of a more severe nature.

Early use of non-steroidal anti-inflammatory medication may be very beneficial in reducing the inflammation occurring in conjunction with soft tissue injury. However, people should be aware of possible side effects from these drugs and only take them on the advice of a medical practitioner.

Children are not just 'young adults'. Sprains and strains in children should not be treated in the same manner as soft tissue injuries in adults. Any child with a limp or not using a limb should be assessed medically to rule out more sinister causes and should not be dismissed with a diagnosis of 'growing pains'.

I am sure this book will soon be a frequently consulted 'reference' on the book shelves of many New Zealand households.

Ruth Highet, MB ChB, Dip. Obs., Dip. Sports Med. (London), FACSP, FASCM

CONTENTS

CHAPTER ONE

INTRODUCTION

Most people, at some stage, have sprained a joint, pulled a muscle or been badly bruised. These so-called soft tissue injuries not only occur to those engaged in sporting activities, but affect people from all walks of life, be it at home, at work or during recreational activity. There are many conflicting remedies for the treatment of these injuries. We are often unsure whether to move or rest the injured area, heat or cool it, rub something into it or leave it alone.

The treatment of soft tissue injuries, whether recent or long-standing, is based on simple principles. An understanding of your injury and your body's repair processes is often all you need to effectively treat your own strains, sprains and bruises.

Who Can Use This Book

This book is for people aged thirteen and older who are in good health. We recommend that children up to the age of thirteen and people with health problems be assessed by a medical practitioner before using this book.

This Book Describes

- The soft tissues of your body that may be injured.
- The types of injuries that may occur.
- How your body responds to injury.
- Treatment principles for recent and long-standing injuries.
- The types of pain experienced at different stages following injury.
- **The most common soft tissue injuries and their treatment.**
- When it is appropriate to seek advice from a doctor or physiotherapist.
- **How to prevent injuries from recurring.**

How To Use This Book

To effectively use this book, it is necessary to **first read chapters one to seven**. Then:

- Refer to the body charts on pages 18 and 19 and locate the site of your injury.
- Turn to the appropriate chapter for your particular injury and *closely* follow the treatment guidelines.
- Read chapters 20 and 21 on injury prevention and stretching exercises to reduce the chances of future injuries.

We hope you will find this book an informative and useful guide for the self-treatment of your strains, sprains and bruises.

We would like to hear from you what aspects of this book you found helpful and more importantly, what you feel could be improved. Please write with your comments to:

Feedback
Treat Your Own Strains, Sprains and Bruises
Spinal Publications
P.O. Box 93
Waikanae
New Zealand

CHAPTER TWO
SOFT TISSUES OF THE BODY

Strains, sprains and bruises affect the soft tissues of the body. Most commonly involved are the joint capsules, ligaments, muscles and tendons. In order to treat soft tissue injuries effectively, a basic understanding of the structure and function of the musculo-skeletal system is required.

We will describe the various bony and soft tissue parts of the body which may be injured and use an illustration of the foot (Fig. 2a) to assist you to identify these structures.

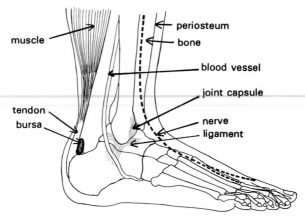

Fig. 2a   Side view of right foot.

Bones And Periosteum

Bones form the rigid framework of the body. Periosteum is the sensitive covering layer of the bone to which the tendons, capsules and ligaments are attached.

Joints, Capsules And Ligaments

Joints are the meeting places of two or more bones where movement takes place. All joints are encased by a tough capsule. Capsules are reinforced by strap-like bands called ligaments. Capsules and ligaments have little 'give' and are common sites for injury.

3

Muscles And Tendons

Muscles are fleshy tissues, richly supplied with blood vessels. They contract and shorten, or relax and lengthen. Tendons are strong cable-like structures, which anchor the muscles to the bone. The muscle-tendon unit is responsible for producing movement at the joints. When compared to muscles, tendons have a poor blood supply and therefore heal at a slower rate.

Bursae

Bursae are fluid-filled sacs, strategically placed to reduce friction between layers of tissues; for example, between tendons and bone.

Nerves

Nerves are the communication lines connecting the brain and spinal cord with the tissues of the body.

Blood Vessels

Blood vessels supply nutrition to and remove waste products from the tissues of the body.

CHAPTER THREE
TYPES OF INJURIES

Soft tissue injuries can be divided into two categories:

1. **Traumatic injuries**
2. **Overuse injuries**

Traumatic Injuries

A traumatic injury occurs instantly as a result of a specific incident. The causes of traumatic injuries are:

— An outside force which comes into contact with the body with sufficient force to cause soft tissue damage; for example, a kick to the shin (Fig. 3a) or a fall onto the shoulder (Fig. 3b).

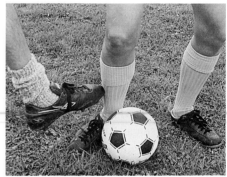

Fig. 3a   Kick to shin.

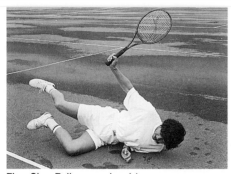

Fig. 3b   Fall onto shoulder.

— A sudden forceful action or unco-ordinated movement which causes overstretching of soft tissues; for example, straining a calf muscle when pushing off for a tennis shot (Fig. 3c).

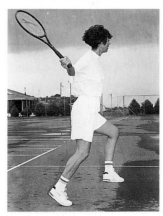

Fig. 3c   Pushing off for tennis shot.

A traumatic injury may affect any of the soft tissues of the body. The injury is called a strain when muscles or tendons are involved. The injury is called a sprain when joint capsules or ligaments are affected. In the event that blood vessels are damaged, internal bleeding will occur and may become visible as bruising.

Overuse Injuries

An overuse injury develops over a period of hours, days or weeks as a result of unaccustomed or excessive, repetitive activities. Examples of repetitive activities are pruning (Fig. 3d), working on a production line, operating a keyboard, or prolonged running (Fig. 3e). The resulting injuries most commonly affect tendons, periosteum, and bone.

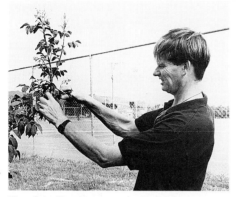

Fig. 3d Pruning.   Fig. 3e   Long distance running.

An overuse injury often begins as a minor irritation in the affected tissues. The pain from such an injury is at first eased by moving the involved area and is therefore often ignored. However, as the tissues become more irritable, the pain becomes worse with work or exercising. Persisting with repetitive activities does not allow the slow-healing tissues to fully repair themselves. If this repeated aggravation is continued and the problem is ignored, a long-term overuse injury will develop which is difficult to self-treat.

There are many underlying causes of overuse injuries. Some of these are:

- A sudden increase or change in activity.
- A lack of general fitness and flexibility.
- Incorrect technique whilst performing an activity.
- Unsuitable equipment or training surfaces.
- Poor design of a work area.

> **The most common causes of overuse injuries are:**
> **too much, too soon, too often.**

This book enables you to treat straightforward overuse injuries. Some overuse injuries do not respond to self-treatment alone. Guidelines are given in each treatment chapter for when to seek advice from a physiotherapist.

CHAPTER FOUR

YOUR BODY'S RESPONSE TO INJURY

Your body's response to injury can be divided into three stages:

1. **Soft tissue damage**
2. **Inflammation**
3. **Repair**

To illustrate what happens during these three stages, we will use a sprained ankle as an example (Figs. 4a, 4b and 4c).

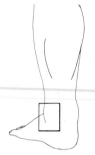

Fig. 4a   Rear view of left ankle.

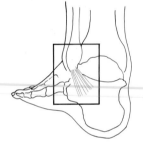

Fig. 4b   Intact ankle ligament.

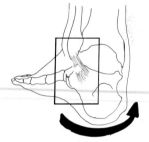

Fig. 4c   Tearing of ankle ligament.

Soft Tissue Damage

Excessive force applied to soft tissues will cause damage. This results in pain and may lead to a certain amount of internal bleeding and swelling (Fig. 4d). Depending on the depth and severity of the injury, a bruise may appear. Bruising is visible evidence that blood vessels have been damaged and blood has seeped out.

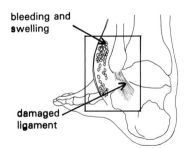

bleeding and swelling

damaged ligament

Fig. 4d   Bleeding and swelling around damaged ligament.

7

Inflammation

Inflammation is your body's first-aid response to injury. It is a localised protective reaction triggered by damage to your soft tissues. Often the inflammatory response is excessive when compared to the actual amount of soft tissue damage. The signs of soft tissue inflammation are: *pain, heat, redness, swelling and loss of movement.* The inflammatory process may continue for five days or more.

If the initial injury is not treated effectively, the inflammatory response can persist for an extended period of time. This may delay repair or lead to a loss of normal flexibility, strength and function following injury.

> **Early and appropriate self-treatment can limit the inflammatory response and enhance recovery.**

Repair

Two to three days after the injury, while the inflammatory response is still taking place, the repair process begins with the formation of new blood vessels around the edge of the injury site. After a further three to five days new tissue is produced. This repair process may continue for several weeks.

The new tissue that is formed is known as *scar tissue* (Fig. 4e). This new tissue does not have the same properties as the original tissue. If not exercised regularly, scar tissue will shrink and shorten. This leads to a reduction in flexibility of the soft tissues and will be felt as pain, stiffness and weakness when attempting to return to normal activity.

> **Scar tissue has the tendency to shrink and shorten.**

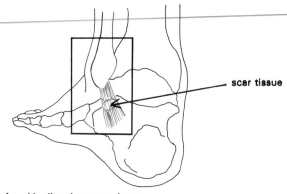

Fig. 4e   Healing by scar tissue.

To avoid the problems described above you must start exercising to stretch and strengthen the healing tissues as soon as possible. Continue the exercises until the injured area has regained its normal flexibility, strength and function. This may take from several weeks to several months, depending on the severity of the injury. Chapter six describes when and how to safely and effectively exercise your injured area.

> **Lack of appropriate exercising is the main reason why soft tissue injuries do not fully recover.**

CHAPTER FIVE

TREATMENT PRINCIPLES
REST, ICE, COMPRESSION, ELEVATION

The regime of *rest, ice, compression and elevation* (RICE) is a simple and effective method of immediate treatment for strains, sprains and bruises. This book also applies the concept of *controlled movement* from the time of injury to full recovery over a period of weeks. Controlled movement is discussed in chapter six.

Rest And Relative Rest

When you feel the pain of an injury, stop whatever you are doing. Use the next few minutes to assess the damage and let the initial pain settle. Then try to move the injured part gently. If the pain becomes worse, you may be increasing the internal bleeding and swelling. To prevent further damage it is necessary to *rest* the injured part for 24 hours. To achieve this you may need to use a walking stick to reduce the weight you take through your injured leg (Fig. 5a) or a sling to support your injured arm.

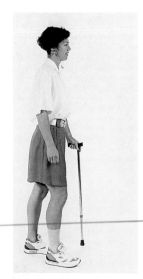

Fig. 5a   Use of walking stick.

When applying the principle of rest following injury it is not necessary to completely stop all activity. The injured part should only be rested to the extent that all painful activities are avoided. This is called *relative rest*. For example, if following an ankle sprain walking does not cause any pain, continue to walk short distances as comfort allows. Maintenance of your general fitness by activities which do not aggravate your injury will assist the early recovery of full function.

Ice And Cold Therapy

Both ice and cold therapy are very effective in reducing inflammation. Ideally, ice or cold therapy should be applied immediately following injury, as this assists to decrease soft tissue damage, pain and muscle spasm.

Ice therapy:

Ice therapy involves the use of ice to obtain cooling of the injured area. The following methods of applying ice are recommended:

- Place crushed ice with a little water in a plastic bag. Then place the bag containing the ice inside another plastic bag and mould this over the injured area.
- Mould a packet of frozen vegetables over the injured area (Fig. 5b).
- Place a commercial therapeutic ice pack on the injured area following the manufacturer's instructions.

Cold therapy:

Cold therapy provides less cooling of the injured area than ice therapy. It is therefore more suitable to apply cold therapy to children, the elderly and persons with a thin, fragile or sensitive skin. The following methods of applying cold therapy are recommended:

- Place a cold, damp flannel over the injured area. The flannel can be cooled by dipping it in ice-water. When the flannel warms up replace it with a cold one.
- Place the injured area in a bucket containing water with a few ice cubes (Fig. 5c). This is useful for foot and hand injuries.
- Place the injured area under cold running water. This is useful for minor injuries or when other options are not available.

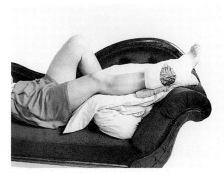

Fig. 5b   Packet of frozen peas.

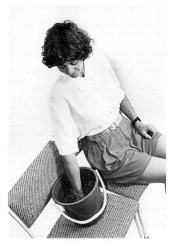

Fig. 5c   A bucket of water with ice cubes.

Guidelines For The Application Of Ice And Cold Therapy

1. **Ice can burn.** To avoid this, protect your skin with a layer of insulation before applying ice therapy. Use a covering of oil, a paper towel or a damp cloth (Fig. 5d). Check your skin after three minutes. If **your skin has become white, stop the ice therapy and use cold therapy instead.**

2. Both ice and cold therapy may give some initial discomfort. This should wear off in a few minutes. If, with the use of *ice* therapy, **your skin is becoming numb or increasingly painful**, stop the ice therapy and use cold therapy instead. If, with the use of *cold* therapy, **your skin is also becoming numb or increasingly painful**, stop the cold therapy and seek advice from a physiotherapist.

3. Apply ice or cold therapy for no longer than 15 minutes. Prolonged application will be of no further benefit.

4. To obtain the maximum benefit, apply ice or cold therapy every three hours. The ideal time to apply ice or cold therapy is after each exercise session.

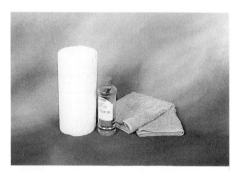

Fig. 5d   Layer of insulation.

Compression

Compression is the application of pressure over the injured area by bandaging (Fig. 5e). This is an invaluable and often overlooked first-aid measure. It is the most effective way of reducing internal bleeding and swelling, particularly if applied within the first few minutes following injury.

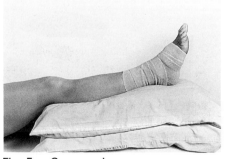

Fig. 5e   Compression.

Guidelines For The Application Of Compression

1. Use a bandage that will mould well around the injured area, providing a firm and even pressure. Elastic bandages are preferable to other types of bandages. Crepe bandages are acceptable but quickly lose their stretch and, consequently, their effectiveness. As an emergency measure, a bed sheet or towel can be torn up and used as a bandage.

2. Bandage a good distance above and below the injury site, working from below upward.

3. Apply the bandage firmly and comfortably. If it is too tight, particularly at night, it may cause pain or numbness. If it is too loose, it will not be effective.

4. Wear the bandage day and night.

5. Remove the bandage before ice or cold therapy and re-apply it immediately afterwards. Re-apply the bandage on rising in the morning and whenever the bandage has become loose or the pressure uneven.

Elevation

Immediately following injury, elevate the injured limb above the level of your heart to limit the development of swelling (Fig. 5f). Elevate your injured limb at every opportunity for as long as the swelling continues. Raising the injured limb above the level of your heart may be impractical at work and in other situations, but remember that some elevation is better than none at all. For example, resting your injured ankle on a chair (Fig. 5g) will still provide effective elevation.

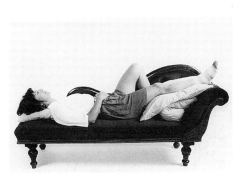

Fig. 5f   Elevation.

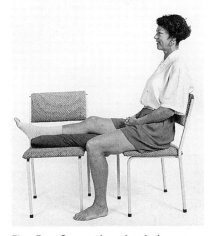

Fig. 5g   Some elevation is better than none at all.

13

Guidelines For When To Apply RICE

1. At the time of injury immediately stop your activity. To prevent further damage, restrict any activity that is painful.

2. Apply ice or cold therapy as soon as possible after the injury has occurred.

3. Apply compression, using a bandage, **immediately** following ice or cold therapy.

4. Elevate your injured area above the level of your heart at regular intervals during the day. This provides an excellent opportunity to apply the ice or cold therapy and compression whilst resting your injury.

5. As your pain and swelling decrease, reduce the application of ice or cold therapy to twice daily. When your daily activities are no longer painful, stop the ice or cold therapy.

6. Continue with compression and regular elevation until the swelling has disappeared. Compare your injured side with the other side to determine whether swelling is present or not.

CHAPTER SIX

TREATMENT PRINCIPLES
CONTROLLED MOVEMENT

In order to restore the normal function of your soft tissues following injury, the concept of controlled movement is used. Controlled movement is the careful exercising of your soft tissues using pain as your guide. The amount and type of exercise to be performed depends on the stage of healing your injury has reached.

**Controlled movement is the careful exercising
of your soft tissues.**

Controlled Movement For A Recent Injury

In the case of a recent soft tissue injury, the injured area needs to be exercised carefully over three to six weeks to ensure a full recovery. This book uses the following regime of controlled movement in each of the treatment chapters:

Two days following the injury careful exercising may be commenced (DAY TWO TO DAY THREE in the treatment chapters). At this stage your injury will be stabilising. Gentle controlled movement that does *not produce or increase pain* at your injury site, stimulates the healing process without causing further damage.

Depending on your progress, four days following the injury the exercises are increased in strength and duration (DAY FOUR TO DAY EIGHT in the treatment chapters). By the fourth day the healing process will have started. Controlled movement that produces *a gentle stretch but no pain* at your injury site, exercises the newly developing scar tissue. This forms the basis for quality healing.

Again, depending on your progress, nine days following the injury the exercises are further increased in strength and duration (DAY NINE TO DAY TWENTY-ONE in the treatment chapters). By the ninth day the healing process will be well established. Controlled movement that produces *a firm stretch but no pain* leads to a strong and flexible repair.

Twenty-two days following the injury your progress is reviewed and injury prevention is discussed (DAY TWENTY-TWO and PREVENTION OF RE-INJURY in the treatment chapters). By the twenty-second day your injury site will have a much improved flexibility, strength and function.

Depending on the extent of your recovery it may be necessary to continue the treatment programme for up to a further three weeks to regain normal function.

Controlled Movement For A Long-Standing Injury

In the case of a long-standing injury, the actual soft tissue damage has healed. *Lack of appropriate exercise* at the time of healing has resulted in a loss of normal flexibility, strength and function. To ensure your long-standing injury has the basis of a stable repair, commence the programme at DAY FOUR TO DAY EIGHT in the treatment chapters. Generally, *long-standing injuries take longer to fully recover than recent injuries* but they respond equally well to the progressions of controlled movement described in this book.

Guidelines For Exercising

1. When commencing an exercise, perform the exercise once, gently and with care, to test the soft tissues involved. The movement may cause discomfort but should not produce or increase pain.

2. Carefully perform the exercise a further three times and evaluate the amount of discomfort caused by these movements.

3. If, on repetition, the exercise only causes discomfort at the extremes of movement, it is safe to continue exercising.

4. If, on repetition, the exercise is painful or constant pain is still felt half an hour after exercising, movement has been applied too early or too vigorously. Continuation of the exercise will disrupt the repair process. Stop exercising and apply RICE. Rest for 24 hours, then begin the exercise again. Perform the exercise more *gently* but just as often.

When performing the exercises described in the treatment programme for your injury, you may feel that one exercise appears to stretch your injury site more than the other exercises. It is necessary to perform every exercise to ensure that all the soft tissues around your injury site regain and maintain their normal flexibility, strength and function.

Appropriate controlled movement leads to a strong and flexible repair.

CHAPTER SEVEN

TYPES OF PAIN

Constant And Intermittent Pain

Pain plays a vital role in the protection of your body and therefore should not be ignored. Identifying whether you are experiencing *constant* or *intermittent* pain will assist you to determine the nature of your problem, the stage of healing you have reached, and the treatment necessary to obtain full recovery. Constant pain is pain that is felt at all times, whether you are active and moving about or at rest. Intermittent pain is pain that is not felt at all times: there will be times in the day that you are completely painfree.

At the time of injury a sharp, localised pain is felt as soft tissues are damaged. After five to ten minutes this sharp, localised pain is followed by a *constant* dull or throbbing pain. This constant pain is caused by the inflammation that is developing in the damaged tissues.

Once the repair process is well on the way, the constant pain will be replaced by an *intermittent* pain. This intermittent pain is felt only when the healing tissues are overstretched. The change from constant to intermittent pain usually takes place two to three days following injury. If healing tissues are re-injured and further soft tissue damage occurs, constant pain will be felt again.

> **Constant pain is pain that is felt at all times.**
> **Intermittent pain is pain that is not felt at all times.**

Referred Pain

Referred pain is pain that is felt at some distance from the actual injury site. If your pain spreads down your arm or leg (Figs. 7a and 7b), it may be referred to that area from your neck or lower back. In addition to the

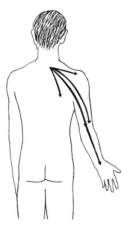

Fig. 7a Common sites of pain referred from neck.

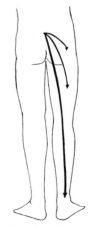

Fig. 7b Common sites of pain referred from lower back.

referred pain you may feel other referred symptoms such as numbness, tingling or pins and needles. If you experience any of these, seek advice from a doctor or physiotherapist.

BODY CHARTS

Locate your injury on the body charts and turn to the appropriate page for self-treatment.

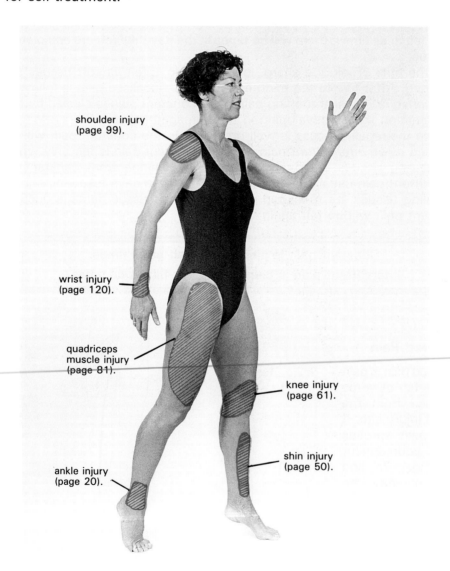

shoulder injury (page 99).

wrist injury (page 120).

quadriceps muscle injury (page 81).

knee injury (page 61).

shin injury (page 50).

ankle injury (page 20).

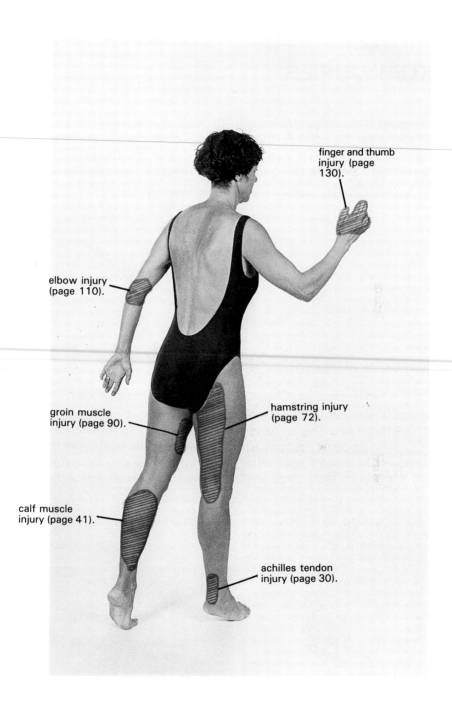

finger and thumb
injury (page
130).

elbow injury
(page 110).

groin muscle
injury (page 90).

hamstring injury
(page 72).

calf muscle
injury (page 41).

achilles tendon
injury (page 30).

CHAPTER EIGHT

ANKLE INJURIES

The design of the ankle enables you to walk and run on flat as well as uneven surfaces. To achieve this the joints of the ankle and foot allow movement in 'up and down' and 'in and out' directions. The ankle therefore relies on strong ligaments and good balance reactions for stability (Fig. 8a).

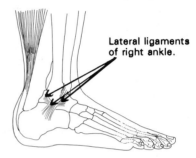

Lateral ligaments of right ankle.

Fig. 8a   Side view of right ankle.

The main cause of injury is:

Traumatic Injury

A traumatic injury commonly involves a sudden twist of (Fig. 8b) or kick to (Fig. 8c) the ankle. The ankle is vulnerable to being sprained by rolling over onto the outside of the foot. The ligaments on the outside of the ankle are more frequently damaged than those on the inside. Repeated minor sprains, if left untreated, may lead to a weak and unstable ankle.

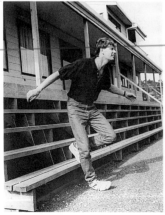

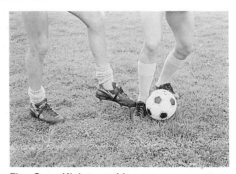

Fig. 8b   Sudden twist of ankle.   Fig. 8c   Kick to ankle.

In a typical ankle injury you will have experienced the following:

Traumatic Injury	
Pain	— At the time of injury a localised sharp pain is felt, usually on the outside of the ankle. This is followed by a constant dull pain. — As the injury heals, the constant pain is replaced by an intermittent pain that is felt only when the soft tissues are overstretched.
Swelling and Bruising	— Swelling frequently develops around the ankle shortly after injury. This may extend into the foot. — Bruising may appear after a few days.
Movement and Activity	Movements and activities limited by pain are: — Pointing the foot down. — Turning the foot in. — Walking, running and hopping.

SERIOUS INJURY

Your injury may be serious when:

a. You are unable to support any weight through your affected leg when attempting to walk one hour after the injury occurred.

b. Substantial swelling appears *within five minutes* of the onset of the injury.

c. Severe pain lasts longer than one hour after the injury occurred.

d. Your pain gets worse over two days or you generally feel unwell.

If **one or more** of the above points apply to you, seek medical advice. In the meantime refer to DAY ONE for the application of RICE to limit further damage. If **none of the above points apply to you, you are an ideal candidate for self-treatment.**

SELF-TREATMENT

If this is the first time you are using this book, **read chapters one to seven before commencing self-treatment.** If your injury happened three days ago or less, start the treatment programme at DAY ONE. If your injury happened more than three days ago, start the treatment programme at DAY FOUR TO DAY EIGHT.

DAY ONE

RICE

Apply rest, ice, compression and elevation every three hours. **Read the guidelines in chapter five (pages 12, 13 and 14) for the safe and effective application of ice and cold therapy, compression and RICE.** Figs. 8d, 8e and 8f demonstrate the application of RICE to your injured ankle.

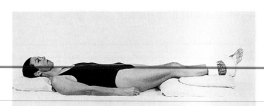

Fig. 8d   Rest, ice and elevation.

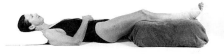

Fig. 8e   Rest, elevation and compression.
Start bandaging at toes, finish well above ankle.

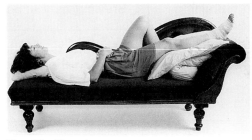

Fig. 8f   Elevation.

Relative Rest

If walking does not cause any pain, continue to walk with care. If walking is painful, rest for 24 hours. The use of a walking stick (Fig. 8g) will help when you have to walk short distances.

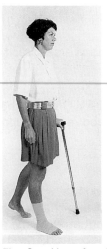

Fig. 8g   Use of walking stick.

DAY TWO

Review your progress

Answer the questions below to review your progress:
- Is your pain intermittent?
- Is your pain constant but less severe than yesterday?
- Are you able to walk short distances with the use of a stick?

If you answer **'yes' to one or more** of the above questions, your ankle injury is improving. Progress to DAY TWO TO DAY THREE of the treatment programme. If you answer **'no' to all** of the above questions, seek advice from a doctor or physiotherapist.

DAY TWO TO DAY THREE

Movement

Even though you may still have constant pain, you may begin to exercise your injured ankle and walk short distances as comfort allows. Try to walk smoothly and with even steps. When exercising, carefully move your ankle. Gentle movement may cause discomfort but should *not produce or increase pain* at your injury site. Perform exercises 8.1 and 8.2 every three hours, following the guidelines for exercising on page 16.

Exercise 8.1   Position yourself as in Fig. 8.1a with your leg resting on a firm surface. *Gently* move your foot up (Fig. 8.1b) and down (Fig. 8.1c) as far as is comfortable. Return to the starting position and perform this exercise four times.

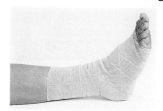 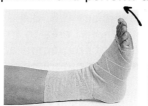 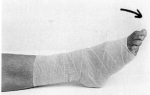

Fig. 8.1a Starting position. Fig. 8.1b Move foot up. Fig. 8.1c Move foot down.

Exercise 8.2   Position yourself as in Fig. 8.2a with your leg resting on a firm surface. *Gently* move your foot in (Fig. 8.2b) and out (Fig. 8.2c) as far as is comfortable. Return to the starting position and perform this exercise four times.

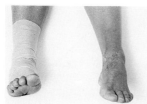 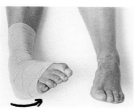 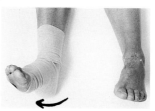

Fig. 8.2a Starting position. Fig. 8.2b Move foot in. Fig. 8.2c Move foot out.

RICE

Apply relative rest, ice, compression and elevation following each exercise session. **Have you read the guidelines in chapter five (pages 12, 13 and 14)?**

DAY FOUR

Review your progress

Answer the questions below to review your progress:

> – Has your pain become intermittent?
> – Do you have less swelling at your injury site?
> – Is there increased movement at your ankle?
> – Is walking more comfortable?

If you answer **'yes' to all** of the above questions, your ankle continues to improve. Progress to DAY FOUR TO DAY EIGHT of the treatment programme. If you answer **'no' to one or more** of the above questions, seek advice from a doctor or physiotherapist.

DAY FOUR TO DAY EIGHT

Start here if your injury is more than three days old

Movement

Gradually increase the exercising of your injured leg. Walk smoothly and with even steps. Perform exercises 8.3, 8.4 and 8.5 every three hours. When exercising move your injured area to the point of *stretch but not pain*. If you started this treatment programme at DAY ONE, stop exercises 8.1 and 8.2. If you are starting the programme now, follow the guidelines for exercising on page 16.

Exercise 8.3   Position yourself as in Fig. 8.3a with your leg resting on a firm surface. Slowly move your foot up until you feel a *gentle stretch* at your injury site (Fig. 8.3b) and hold for one second. Then slowly move your foot down until you feel a *gentle stretch* at your injury site (Fig. 8.3c) and hold for one second. Return to the starting position and perform this exercise four times.

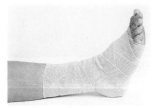

Fig. 8.3a   Starting position.

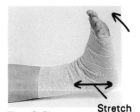

Fig. 8.3b.   Stretch

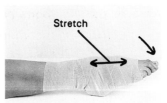

Fig. 8.3c.

Exercise 8.4   Position yourself as in Fig. 8.4a with your leg resting on a firm surface. Slowly move your foot in until you feel a *gentle stretch* at your injury site (Fig. 8.4b) and hold for one second. Then slowly move your foot out until you feel a *gentle stretch* at your injury site (Fig. 8.4c) and hold for one second. Return to the starting position and perform this exercise four times. Keep your leg still to ensure these movements occur only at the ankle.

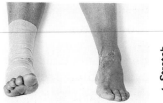

Fig. 8.4a   Starting position.   Fig. 8.4b.   Fig 8.4c.

Exercise 8.5   Stand close to a chair, table, or wall for support. Balance on your injured foot (Fig. 8.5a) for up to 10 seconds. Perform this exercise four times.

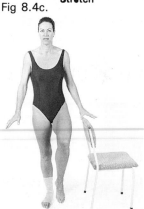

Fig. 8.5a   Balance.

RICE

Continue with the application of relative rest, ice, compression and elevation following each exercise session. If you are starting the programme now, **refer to DAY ONE — 'RICE' and 'Relative rest' — of this treatment chapter (page 22).** Figs. 8d, 8e and 8f demonstrate the application of RICE to your injured ankle.

DAY NINE

Review your progress

Answer the questions below to review your progress:

- Do you have intermittent pain only when overstretching the injured area?
- Do you have little or no swelling at your injury site?
- Are you able to perform exercises 8.3, 8.4 and 8.5 without difficulty?
- Can you walk without limping?

If you answer **'yes' to all** of the above questions, your injury continues to improve. Progress to DAY NINE TO DAY TWENTY-ONE of the treatment programme. If you answer **'no' to one or more** of the above questions, seek advice from a doctor or physiotherapist.

DAY NINE TO DAY TWENTY-ONE

Movement

Return to your daily activities as comfort allows. Do not attempt to run until you can walk on your tiptoes and hop several times without pain. Regain and maintain your general fitness by activities that are unlikely to aggravate your injury; for example, swimming or cycling. Stop exercises 8.3, 8.4 and 8.5. Perform exercises 8.6, 8.7, 8.8 and 8.9 every three hours. When exercising move your injured ankle to the point of *firm stretch but not pain*, following the guidelines for exercising on page 16.

Exercise 8.6   Position yourself as in Fig. 8.6a. Taking your weight through your hands, slowly lower yourself onto your heels until you feel a *firm stretch* at your injury site (Fig. 8.6b) and hold for three seconds. Return to the starting position and perform this exercise four times. As your injury improves, take less weight through your hands until you no longer require support (Fig. 8.6c). If you have a knee problem, do not attempt this exercise. Continue with exercise 8.3, but move your ankle until you feel a *firm stretch* at your injury site and hold for three seconds. Perform this exercise four times.

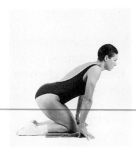
Fig. 8.6a   Starting position.

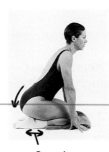
Stretch
Fig 8.6b.

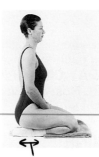
Stretch
Fig 8.6c.

Exercise 8.7   Position yourself as in Fig. 8.7a. Taking most of the weight through your uninjured leg, slowly roll over onto the outside of your injured foot until you feel a *firm stretch* at your injury site (Fig. 8.7b) and hold for three seconds. Return to the starting position and perform this exercise four times. As your injury improves you will be able to take more weight through your injured leg.

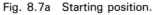

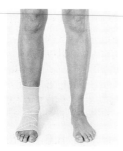 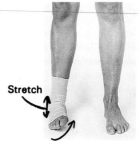

Fig. 8.7a   Starting position.   Fig. 8.7b.

Exercise 8.8   Position yourself as in Fig. 8.8a and 8.8b with your feet parallel and your injured leg behind. Bend your rear knee and ankle, keeping your heels on the ground. Slowly bend further until you feel a *firm stretch* at your injury site (Fig. 8.8c) and hold for three seconds. Return to the starting position and perform this exercise four times.

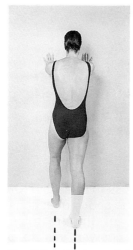 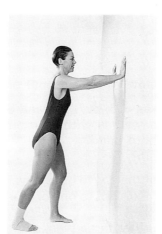 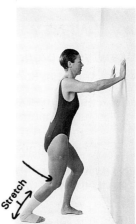

Fig. 8.8a   Feet parallel.   Fig. 8.8b   Starting position.   Fig. 8.8c.

Exercise 8.9   Stand close to a chair, table or wall for support. Balance
                on your injured foot (Fig. 8.9a) for up to 30 seconds. Once
                every ten seconds carefully rise up on your toes (Fig.
                8.9b) and ease down whilst maintaining your balance.
                Perform this exercise four times.

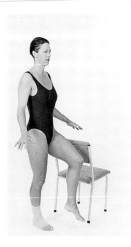

Fig. 8.9a   Balance.

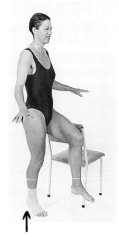

Fig. 8.9b   Rise up on toes.

RICE

As your pain and swelling decrease, you may reduce the number of times
you apply RICE. **Read the guidelines in chapter five (page 14) for when
to apply RICE.**

DAY TWENTY-TWO

Review your progress

Answer the questions below to review your progress. Are you able to:

-    Perform exercises 8.6, 8.7, 8.8 and 8.9 with your injured
     ankle almost as well as with your uninjured ankle?
-    Jog or run without pain?
-    Hop without pain?

If you answer **'yes' to all** of the above questions, progress to PREVENTION
OF RE-INJURY. If you answer **'no' to one or more** of the above questions,
continue with DAY NINE TO DAY TWENTY-ONE of the treatment
programme for up to a further three weeks until you answer **'yes' to all**
of the above questions. If, after three weeks, you still answer **'no' to one
or more** of the above questions, seek advice from a physiotherapist.

PREVENTION OF RE-INJURY

Read chapters 20 and 21 on injury prevention and stretching exercises.

If your work or recreational activities involve running or jumping, a gradual build-up over three weeks is essential. This allows your ankle to fully regain the ability to perform these more demanding tasks without the danger of re-injury.

If your ankle feels unstable when walking on uneven ground, running or jumping, strapping may be required for additional support. Seek advice on strapping from a physiotherapist.

CHAPTER NINE

ACHILLES TENDON INJURIES

The achilles tendon is the prominent tendon just above the back of the heel attaching the calf muscles to the foot (Fig. 9a). This muscle-tendon unit plays a vital role in the 'pushing-off' action necessary for walking and running. Injury to the achilles tendon leads to a condition called 'achilles tendinitis'. This is an inflammation of the tendon or its covering layer.

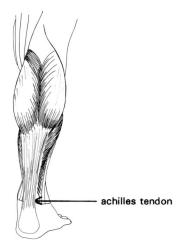

achilles tendon

Fig. 9a   Rear view of right leg.

The two main causes of injury are:

Traumatic Injury

A traumatic injury commonly involves a strain or partial tearing of the tendon, often caused by an unexpected stretch; for example, an unco-ordinated lunge or leap during sport (Fig. 9b). The achilles tendon can also be injured by a direct blow; for example, being hit by a supermarket trolley.

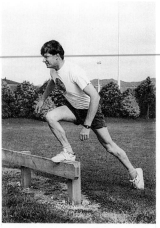

Fig. 9b   Unco-ordinated leap.

Overuse Injury

An overuse injury involves an inflammation of the tendon or its covering layer from unaccustomed or excessive, repetitive activity; for example, long distance running (Fig. 9c), the first tramp or hike of the season, or aerobics. Contributing factors which may lead to overuse injury are:

- Repetitive jumping or other high impact activities.
- Worn-out or inappropriate footwear.
- A sudden increase or change in training activities.
- An abnormal alignment of the joints in the foot.
- Tight calf muscles.

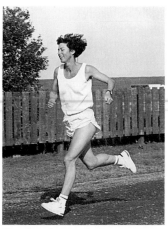

Fig. 9c   Long distance running.

In the early stages the pain eases with activity and the problem is often ignored. Continuing the activity results in a long-standing overuse injury. This type of injury can take considerable time to heal and may be difficult to self-treat.

In a typical achilles tendon injury you will have experienced the following:

	Traumatic Injury	Overuse Injury
Pain	– At the time of injury a localised sharp pain is felt just above the heel. This is followed by a constant dull pain. – As the injury heals, the constant pain is replaced by an intermittent pain that is felt only when the soft tissues are over-stretched.	– In the early stages pain is felt before and after activity but eases during exercise. – Continued aggravation of the overuse injury leads to a constant dull or throbbing pain.
Swelling and Bruising	Swelling frequently develops around the achilles tendon shortly after injury.	Swelling often develops around the achilles tendon if the overuse activity is continued.
Movement and Activity	Movements and activities limited by pain are: – Pulling the foot up. – Walking. – Standing on tiptoes. – Hopping, jumping and running.	– Some stiffness is experienced when beginning activity after resting or sleeping. – Full movement of the ankle is usually present.

SERIOUS INJURY

Your injury may be serious when:

a. You are unable to support any weight through your affected leg when attempting to walk one hour after the injury occurred.

b. You cannot put your heel on the ground when attempting to walk 24 hours after the injury occurred.

c. You are unable to rise up on the toes of your affected leg 48 hours after the injury occurred.

d. Your pain gets worse over two days or you generally feel unwell.

If **one or more** of the above points apply to you, seek medical advice. In the meantime refer to DAY ONE for the application of RICE to limit further damage. If **none of the above points apply to you, you are an ideal candidate for self-treatment.**

SELF-TREATMENT

If this is the first time you are using this book, **read chapters one to seven before commencing self-treatment.** If your injury happened three days ago or less, start the treatment programme at DAY ONE. If your injury happened more than three days ago, start the treatment programme at DAY FOUR TO DAY EIGHT.

DAY ONE
RICE

Apply rest, ice, compression and elevation every three hours. **Read the guidelines in chapter five (pages 12, 13 and 14) for the safe and effective application of ice and cold therapy, compression and RICE.** Figs. 9d and 9e demonstrate the application of RICE to your injured achilles tendon.

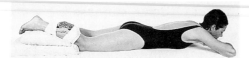

Fig. 9d   Rest, ice and elevation.

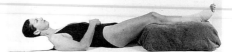

Fig. 9e   Rest, elevation and compression. Start bandaging at toes, finish well above ankle.

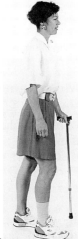

Relative rest

If walking does not cause any pain, continue to walk with care. If walking is painful, rest for 24 hours. The use of a walking stick (Fig. 9f) will help when you have to walk short distances.

Fig. 9f
Use of walking stick.

Use a heel raise to ease the stress on your achilles tendon. There are various ways to raise your heel. You may wear shoes with a 2 to 3 cm heel or insert a heel raise into a flat shoe. You can buy a commercial heel raise, insert a piece of carpet cut to your heel size, or use two folded handkerchiefs (Fig. 9g).

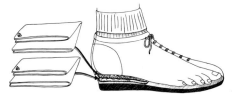

Fig. 9g   Insert two folded handkerchiefs.

DAY TWO

Review your progress

Answer the questions below to review your progress:

- Is your pain intermittent?
- Is your pain constant but less severe than yesterday?
- Are you able to walk short distances with the use of a stick?

If you answer **'yes' to one or more** of the above questions, your achilles tendon injury is improving. Progress to DAY TWO TO DAY THREE of the treatment programme. If you answer **'no' to all** of the above questions, seek advice from a doctor or physiotherapist.

DAY TWO TO DAY THREE

Movement

You may begin to exercise your injured leg and walk short distances as comfort allows. Try to walk smoothly and with even steps. When exercising, carefully move your foot. Gentle movement may cause discomfort but should *not produce or increase pain* at your injury site. Perform exercise 9.1 every three hours, following the guidelines for exercising on page 16.

Exercise 9.1   Position yourself as in Fig. 9.1a with your leg resting on a firm surface. *Gently* move your foot up (Fig. 9.1b) and down (Fig. 9.1c) as far as is comfortable. Return to the starting position and perform this exercise four times.

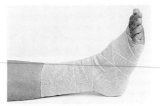
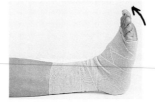
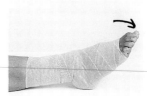

Fig. 9.1a Starting position.   Fig. 9.1b   Fig. 9.1c

RICE

Apply relative rest, ice, compression and elevation following each exercise session. **Have you read the guidelines in chapter five (pages 12, 13 and 14)?**

DAY FOUR

Review your progress

Answer the questions below to review your progress:

- Has your pain become intermittent?
- Is there increased movement at your ankle?
- Is walking more comfortable?

If you answer **'yes' to all** of the above questions, your achilles tendon continues to improve. Progress to DAY FOUR TO DAY EIGHT of the treatment programme. If you answer **'no' to one or more** of the above questions, seek advice from a doctor or physiotherapist.

DAY FOUR TO DAY EIGHT

Start here if your injury is more than three days old

Movement

Gradually increase the exercising of your injured achilles tendon. Walk smoothly and with even steps. Perform exercises 9.2 and 9.3 every three hours. When exercising move your injured area to the point of *stretch but not pain*. If you started this treatment programme at DAY ONE, stop exercise 9.1. If you are starting the programme now, follow the guidelines for exercising on page 16.

Exercise 9.2 Position yourself as in Figs. 9.2a and 9.2b with your feet parallel and a shoulder-width apart. Keeping your knees straight and heels on the ground, slowly lean forward until you feel a *gentle stretch* at your injury site (Fig. 9.2c) and hold for five seconds. Return to the starting position and perform this exercise four times.

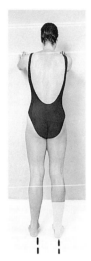

Fig. 9.2a Feet parallel.

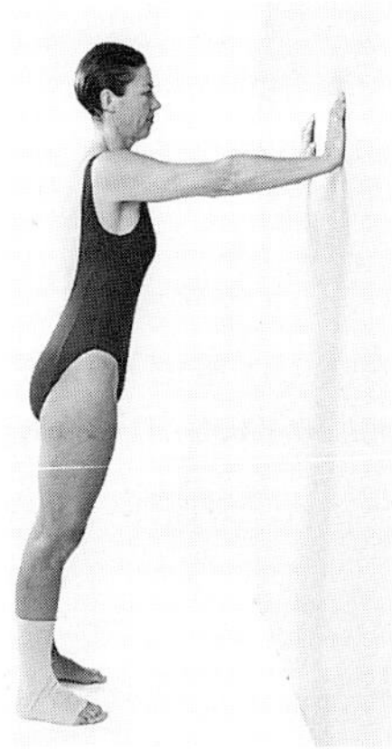

Fig. 9.2b Starting position.

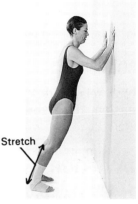

Fig. 9.2c

Exercise 9.3 Position yourself as in Figs. 9.3a and 9.3b with your feet parallel and a shoulder-width apart. Keeping your heels on the ground, slowly bend at your knees and ankles until you feel a *gentle stretch* at your injury site (Fig. 9.3c) and hold for five seconds. Return to the starting position and perform this exercise four times.

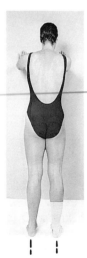

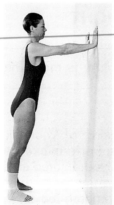

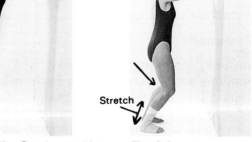

Fig. 9.3a Feet parallel.

Fig. 9.3b Starting position.

Fig. 9.3c

RICE

Continue with the application of relative rest, ice, compression and elevation following each exercise session. If you are starting the programme now, **refer to DAY ONE—'RICE' and 'Relative rest'—of this treatment chapter (page 33).** Figs. 9d, 9e and 9g demonstrate the application of RICE to your injured achilles tendon and the use of a heel raise.

DAY NINE

Review your progress

Answer the questions below to review your progress:

- Do you have intermittent pain only when overstretching your injured area?
- Do you have little or no swelling at your injury site?
- Are you able to perform exercises 9.2 and 9.3 without difficulty?
- Can you walk without limping?

If you answer **'yes' to all** of the above questions, your injury continues to improve. Progress to DAY NINE TO DAY TWENTY-ONE of the treatment programme. If you answer **'no' to one or more** of the above questions, seek advice from a doctor or physiotherapist.

DAY NINE TO DAY TWENTY-ONE

Movement

Return to your daily activities as comfort allows. Do not attempt to run until you can walk briskly without experiencing pain or stiffness. Regain and maintain your general fitness by activities that are unlikely to aggravate your injury; for example, swimming or cycling. Continue to use a heel raise or to wear shoes with a raised heel. Stop exercises 9.2 and 9.3. Perform exercises 9.4, 9.5 and 9.6 every three hours. When exercising move the injured area to the point of *firm stretch but not pain*, following the guidelines for exercising on page 16.

Exercise 9.4 Position yourself as in Fig. 9.4a and 9.4b with your feet parallel and your injured leg behind. Lean forward, keeping your rear knee straight and your heels on the ground. Slowly lean further forward until you feel a *firm stretch* at your injury site (Fig. 9.4c) and hold for ten seconds. Return to the starting position and perform this exercise four times.

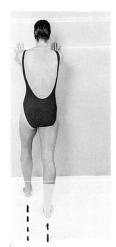

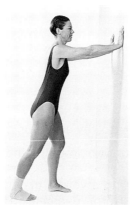

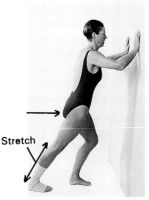

Fig. 9.4a   Feet parallel.   Fig. 9.4b   Starting position.   Fig. 9.4c

Exercise 9.5 Position yourself as in Fig. 9.5a and 9.5b with your feet parallel and your injured leg behind. Bend your rear knee and ankle, keeping your heels on the ground. Slowly bend further until you feel a *firm stretch* at your injury site (Fig. 9.5c) and hold for ten seconds. Return to the starting position and perform this exercise four times.

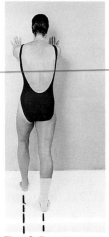

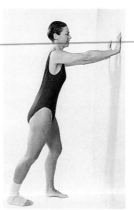

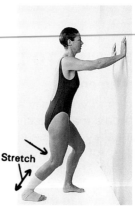

Fig. 9.5a   Feet parallel.   Fig. 9.5b   Starting position.   Fig. 9.5c

Exercise 9.6   Position yourself as in Fig. 9.6a with your heels over the edge of the step and holding onto the wall for support. Taking some of your weight through your injured leg, slowly rise on to your toes (Fig. 9.6b) and hold for five seconds. Then slowly lower yourself until you feel a *firm stretch* at your injury site (Fig. 9.6c) and hold for five seconds. Return to the starting position and perform this exercise four times. As your injury improves, you will be able to take more weight through your injured leg.

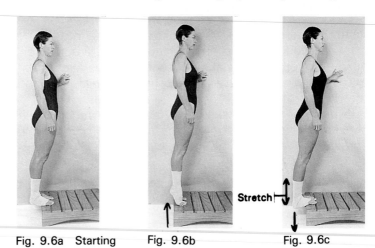

Fig. 9.6a Starting position.   Fig. 9.6b   Fig. 9.6c

RICE

As your pain and swelling decrease, you may reduce the number of times you apply RICE. **Read the guidelines in chapter five (page 14) for when to apply RICE.**

DAY TWENTY-TWO

Review your progress

Answer the questions below to review your progress. Are you able to:

- Perform exercises 9.4, 9.5 and 9.6 with your injured achilles tendon almost as well as with your uninjured achilles tendon?
- Jog or run without pain?
- Hop without pain?

If you answer **'yes' to all** of the above questions, progress to PREVENTION OF RE-INJURY. If you answer **'no' to one or more** of the above questions, continue with DAY NINE TO DAY TWENTY-ONE of the treatment programme and the use of a heel raise for up to a further three weeks until you answer **'yes' to all** of the above questions. If, after three weeks, you still answer **'no' to one or more** of the above questions, seek advice from a physiotherapist.

PREVENTION OF RE-INJURY

Read chapters 20 and 21 on injury prevention and stretching exercises.

If your work or recreational activities involve running or jumping, a gradual build-up over three weeks is essential. This allows your achilles tendon to fully regain the ability to perform these more demanding tasks without the danger of re-injury.

If despite these measures your injury recurs, seek advice from a physiotherapist to determine whether other factors are contributing to this condition.

CHAPTER TEN

CALF MUSCLE INJURIES

The calf consists of two main muscles, one of which originates from above and the other from below the knee joint. These muscles blend to form the achilles tendon which attaches to the back of the heel (Fig. 10a). This muscle-tendon unit plays a vital role in the pushing-off action necessary for walking, running and jumping.

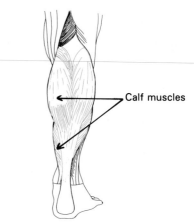

Calf muscles

Fig. 10a   Rear view of right leg.

The main cause of injury is:
Traumatic Injury

A traumatic injury involves a strain of the muscle fibres caused by a sudden forceful action, or a bruise caused by a direct blow; for example, pushing off when running for a tennis shot (Fig. 10b) or a kick to the calf (Fig. 10c).

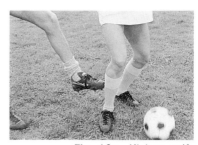

Fig. 10b   Pushing off.

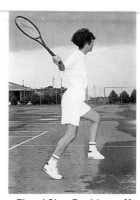

Fig. 10c   Kick to calf.

In a typical calf muscle injury you will have experienced the following:

Traumatic Injury	
Pain	– At the time of the injury a localised sharp pain is felt in the calf. This is followed by a constant dull pain. – As the injury heals, the constant pain is replaced by an intermittent pain that is felt only when the soft tissues are overstretched.
Swelling and Bruising	– Swelling frequently develops in the calf muscles shortly after injury. – After a few days bruising may appear.
Movement and Activity	Movements and activities limited by pain are: – Pulling the foot up. – Walking. – Standing on tiptoes. – Hopping, running and jumping.

SERIOUS INJURY

Your injury may be serious when:

    a.   You are unable to support any weight through your affected leg when attempting to walk one hour after the injury occurred.

    b.   You cannot put your heel on the ground when attempting to walk 48 hours after the injury occurred.

    c.   You are unable to rise on the toes of the affected leg 48 hours after the injury occurred.

    d.   Your pain gets worse over two days or you generally feel unwell.

If **one or more** of the above points apply to you, seek medical advice. In the meantime refer to DAY ONE for the application of RICE to limit further damage. If **none of the above points apply to you, you are an ideal candidate for self-treatment.**

SELF-TREATMENT

If this is the first time you are using this book, **read chapters one to seven before commencing self-treatment.** If your injury happened three days ago or less, start the treatment programme at DAY ONE. If your injury happened more than three days ago, start the treatment programme at DAY FOUR TO DAY EIGHT.

DAY ONE

RICE

Apply rest, ice, compression and elevation every three hours. **Read the guidelines in chapter five (pages 12, 13 and 14) for the safe and effective application of ice and cold therapy, compression and RICE.** Figs. 10d and 10e demonstrate the application of RICE to your injured calf muscle.

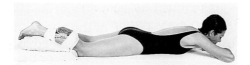

Fig. 10d   Rest, ice and elevation.

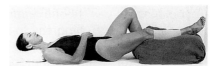

Fig. 10e   Rest, elevation and compression. Start bandaging just above ankle, finish just below knee.

Relative rest

If walking does not cause any pain, continue to walk with care. If walking is painful, rest for 24 hours. The use of a walking stick (Fig. 10f) will help when you have to walk short distances.

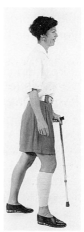

Fig. 10f   Use of walking stick

Use a heel raise to ease the stress on your calf muscle. There are various ways to raise your heel. You may wear shoes with a 2 to 3 cm heel or insert a heel raise into a flat shoe. You can buy a commercial heel raise, insert a small piece of carpet cut to your heel size, or use two folded handkerchiefs (Fig. 10g).

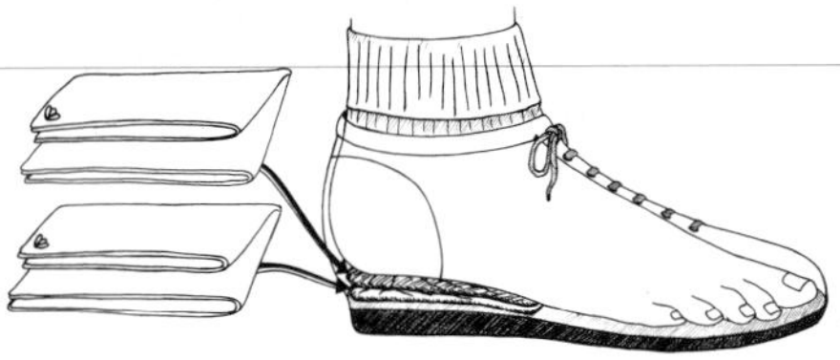

Fig. 10g   Insert two folded handkerchiefs.

DAY TWO
Review your progress

Answer the questions below to review your progress:

- Is your pain intermittent?
- Is your pain constant but less severe than yesterday?
- Are you able to walk short distances with the use of a stick?

If you answer **'yes' to one or more** of the above questions, your calf muscle injury is improving. Progress to DAY TWO TO DAY THREE of the treatment programme. If you answer **'no' to all** of the above questions, seek advice from a doctor or physiotherapist.

DAY TWO TO DAY THREE
Movement

You may begin to exercise your injured calf muscle and walk short distances as comfort allows. Try to walk smoothly and with even steps. When exercising, carefully move your foot. Gentle movement may cause discomfort but should *not produce or increase pain* at your injury site. Perform exercise 10.1 every three hours, following the guidelines for exercising on page 16.

Exercise 10.1   Position yourself as in Fig. 10.1a with your leg resting on a firm surface. *Gently* move your foot up (Fig. 10.1b) and down (Fig. 10.1c) as far as is comfortable. Return to the starting position and perform this exercise four times.

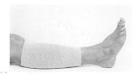
Fig. 10.1a   Starting position.

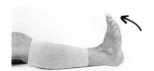
Fig. 10.1b

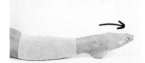
Fig. 10.1c

RICE

Apply relative rest, ice, compression and elevation following each exercise session. **Have you read the guidelines in chapter five (pages 12, 13 and 14)?**

DAY FOUR

Review your progress

Answer the questions below to review your progress:

- Has your pain become intermittent?
- Do you have less swelling at your injury site?
- Is there increased movement at your ankle?
- Is walking more comfortable?

If you answer **'yes' to all** of the above questions, your calf muscle continues to improve. Progress to DAY FOUR TO DAY EIGHT of the treatment programme. If you answer **'no' to one or more** of the above questions, seek advice from a doctor or physiotherapist.

DAY FOUR TO DAY EIGHT

Start here if your injury is more than three days old

Movement

Gradually increase the exercising of your injured calf muscle. Walk smoothly and with even steps. Perform exercises 10.2 and 10.3 every three hours. When exercising move your injured area to the point of *stretch but not pain*. If you started this treatment programme at DAY ONE, stop exercise 10.1. If you are starting the programme now, follow the guidelines for exercising on page 16.

Exercise 10.2   Position yourself as in Fig. 10.2a and 10.2b with your feet parallel and a shoulder-width apart. Slowly lean forward keeping your knees straight and heels on the ground until you feel a *gentle stretch* at your injury site (Fig. 10.2c) and hold for five seconds. Return to the starting position and perform this exercise four times.

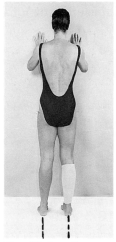
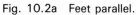
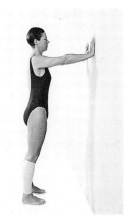
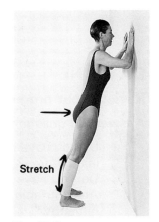

Fig. 10.2a Feet parallel.   Fig. 10.2b Starting position.   Fig. 10.2c

Stretch

Exercise 10.3   Position yourself as in Fig. 10.3a and 10.3b with your feet parallel and a shoulder-width apart. Keeping your heels on the ground, slowly bend at your knees and ankles until you feel a *gentle stretch* at your injury site (Fig. 10.3c) and hold for five seconds. Return to the starting position and perform this exercise four times.

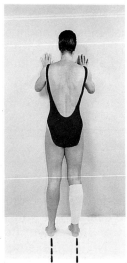
Fig. 10.3a   Feet parallel.

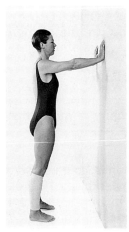
Fig. 10.3b   Starting position.

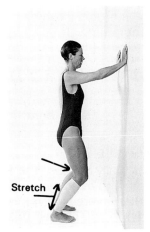
Fig. 10.3c

RICE

Continue with the application of relative rest, ice, compression and elevation following each exercise session. If you are starting the programme now, **refer to DAY ONE—'RICE' and 'Relative rest'—of this treatment chapter (page 43).** Figs. 10d, 10e and 10g demonstrate the application of RICE to your injured calf muscle and the use of a heel raise.

DAY NINE

Review your progress

Answer the questions below to review your progress:

- Do you have intermittent pain only when overstretching your injured area?
- Do you have little or no swelling at your injury site?
- Are you able to perform exercises 10.2 and 10.3 without difficulty?
- Can you walk without limping?

If you answer **'yes' to all** of the above questions, your injury continues to improve. Progress to DAY NINE TO DAY TWENTY-ONE of the treatment programme. If you answer **'no' to one or more** of the above questions, seek advice from a doctor or physiotherapist.

DAY NINE TO DAY TWENTY-ONE
Movement

Return to your daily activities as comfort allows. Do not attempt to run until you can comfortably walk on your tiptoes and hop several times without pain. Regain and maintain your general fitness by activities that are unlikely to aggravate your injury; for example, swimming or cycling. If walking on bare feet still causes discomfort, continue to use a heel raise or to wear shoes with a raised heel. Stop exercises 10.2 and 10.3. Perform exercises 10.4, 10.5 and 10.6 every three hours. When exercising move the injured area to the point of *firm stretch but not pain*, following the guidelines for exercising on page 16.

Exercise 10.4   Position yourself as in Fig. 10.4a and 10.4b with your feet parallel and your injured leg behind. Lean forward, keeping your rear knee straight and your heels on the ground. Slowly lean further forward until you feel a *firm stretch* at your injury site (Fig. 10.4c) and hold for ten seconds. Return to the starting position and perform this exercise four times.

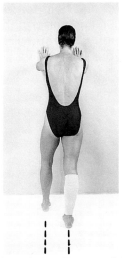 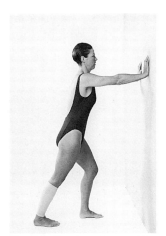 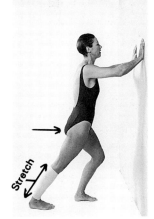

Fig. 10.4a Feet parallel.   Fig. 10.4b Starting position.   Fig. 10.4c

Exercise 10.5   Position yourself as in Fig. 10.5a and 10.5b with your feet parallel and your injured leg behind. Bend your rear knee and ankle, keeping your heels on the ground. Slowly bend further until you feel a *firm stretch* at your injury site (Fig. 10.5c) and hold for ten seconds. Return to the starting position and perform this exercise four times.

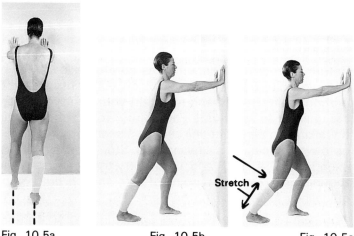

Fig. 10.5a
Feet parallel.

Fig. 10.5b
Starting position.

Fig. 10.5c

Exercise 10.6   Position yourself as in Fig. 10.6a with your heels over the edge of the step and holding onto the wall for support. Taking some of your weight through your injured leg, slowly rise on to your toes (Fig. 10.6b) and hold for five seconds. Then slowly lower yourself until you feel a *firm stretch* at your injury site (Fig. 10.6c) and hold for five seconds. Return to the starting position and perform this exercise four times. As your injury improves, you will be able to take more weight through your injured leg.

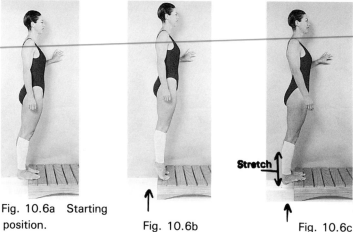

Fig. 10.6a Starting position.

Fig. 10.6b

Fig. 10.6c

RICE

As your pain and swelling decrease, you may reduce the number of times you apply RICE. **Read the guidelines in chapter five (page 14) for when to apply RICE.**

DAY TWENTY-TWO

Review your progress

Answer the questions below to review your progress. Are you able to:

- Perform exercises 10.4, 10.5 and 10.6 with your injured calf muscle almost as well as with your uninjured calf muscle?
- Jog or run without pain?
- Hop without pain?

If you answer **'yes' to all** of the above questions, progress to PREVENTION OF RE-INJURY. If you answer **'no' to one or more** of the above questions, continue with DAY NINE TO DAY TWENTY-ONE of the treatment programme and the use of a heel raise for up to a further three weeks until you answer **'yes' to all** of the above questions. If, after three weeks, you still answer **'no' to one or more** of the above questions, seek advice from a physiotherapist.

PREVENTION OF RE-INJURY

Read chapters 20 and 21 on injury prevention and stretching exercises.

If your work or recreational activities involve running or jumping, a gradual build-up over three weeks is essential. This allows your calf muscle to fully regain the ability to perform these more demanding tasks without the danger of re-injury.

CHAPTER ELEVEN

SHIN INJURIES

The tibia or shin bone has groups of long thin muscles running down either side of it, called the tibial muscles (Fig. 11a). These muscles play an important role in controlling movements of the feet and toes.

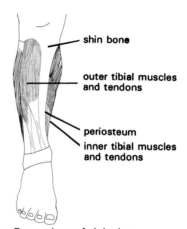

shin bone

outer tibial muscles and tendons

periosteum
inner tibial muscles and tendons

Fig. 11a   Front view of right leg.

The two main causes of injury are:

Traumatic Injury

A traumatic unjury involves either a kick (Fig. 11b) or a direct blow to the shin, resulting in a painful bruising of the bone, periosteum and muscles on either side of the shin.

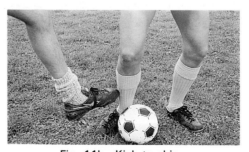

Fig. 11b   Kick to shin.

Overuse Injury

An overuse injury involves an inflammation of the muscles, tendons and periosteum in the lower leg due to unaccustomed or excessive, repetitive activities; for example, tramping, jogging or aerobics (Fig. 11c). The pain is usually felt along the inner side of the shin bone, but may also occur on the outer side. This condition is commonly known as shin splints. Contributing factors which may lead to overuse injury are:

- Repetitive jumping or other high impact activities.
- Worn-out or inappropriate foot wear.
- A sudden increase or change in training activities.
- An abnormal alignment of the joints in the foot.
- Tight calf muscles.

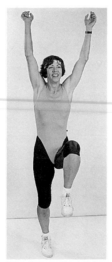

Fig. 11c   Aerobics.

In the early stages the pain eases with activity and the problem is often ignored. Continuing the activity results in a long-standing overuse injury. This type of injury can take considerable time to heal and may be difficult to self-treat.

In a typical shin injury you will have experienced the following:

	Traumatic Injury	Overuse Injury
Pain	− At the time of injury a localised sharp pain is felt. This is followed by a constant dull pain. − As the injury heals, the constant pain is replaced by an intermittent pain that is felt only when the soft tissues are overstretched.	− In the early stages pain is felt before and after activity but eases during exercise. − Continued aggravation of the overuse injury leads to a constant dull or throbbing pain.
Swelling and Bruising	− Swelling frequently develops around the shin shortly after injury. − Bruising may appear after a few days.	Swelling may be present if the injury is severe.
Movement and Activity	Movements and activities limited by pain are: − Pulling the foot and toes up. − Pushing the foot and toes down.	− Stiffness may be felt when beginning activity after resting or sleeping. − Full movement of ankle and foot is usually present.

SERIOUS INJURY

Your injury may be serious when:

a.   You have severe pain or swelling on either side of your shin which does not ease with rest.

b.   The foot of your injured leg feels numb or cold compared to the other side.

c.   You are unable to rise on the toes of the injured leg 24 hours after the injury occurred.

d.   Your pain gets worse over two days or you generally feel unwell.

If **one or more** of the above points apply to you, seek medical advice. In the meantime refer to DAY ONE for the application of RICE to limit further damage. If **none of the above points apply to you, you are an ideal candidate for self-treatment.**

SELF-TREATMENT

If this is the first time you are using this book, **read chapters one to seven before commencing self-treatment.** If your injury happened three days ago or less, start the treatment programme at DAY ONE. If your injury happened more than three days ago, start the treatment programme at DAY FOUR TO DAY EIGHT.

DAY ONE

RICE

Apply rest, ice, compression and elevation every three hours. **Read the guidelines in chapter five (pages 12, 13 and 14) for the safe and effective application of ice and cold therapy, compression and RICE.** Figs. 11d and 11e demonstrate the application of RICE to your injured shin.

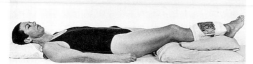

Fig. 11d   Rest, ice and elevation.

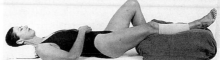

Fig. 11e   Rest, elevation and compression. Start bandaging just above ankle, finish just below knee.

Relative rest

If walking does not cause any pain, continue to walk with care. If walking is painful, rest for 24 hours. The use of a walking stick (Fig. 11f) will help when you have to walk short distances.

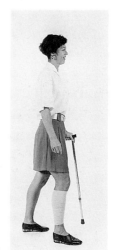

Fig. 11f
Use of walking stick.

DAY TWO

Review your progress

Answer the questions below to review your progress:

- Is your pain intermittent?
- Is your pain constant but less severe than yesterday?
- Are you able to walk short distances with the use of a stick?

If you answer **'yes' to one or more** of the above questions, your shin injury is improving. Progress to DAY TWO TO DAY THREE of the treatment programme. If you answer **'no' to all** of the above questions, seek advice from a doctor or physiotherapist.

DAY TWO TO DAY THREE

Movement

You may begin to exercise your injured shin and walk short distances as comfort allows. Try to walk smoothly and with even steps. When exercising, carefully move your foot. Gentle movement may cause discomfort but should *not produce or increase pain* at your injury site. Perform exercises 11.1 and 11.2 every three hours, following the guidelines on page 16.

Exercise 11.1   Position yourself as in Fig. 11.1a with your leg resting on a firm surface. *Gently* move your foot up (Fig. 11.1b) and down (Fig. 11.1c) as far as is comfortable. Return to the starting position and perform this exercise four times.

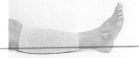
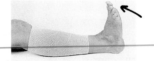

Fig. 11.1a
Starting position.

Fig. 11.1b.

Fig. 11.1c.

Exercise 11.2   Position yourself as in Fig. 11.2a with your leg resting on a firm surface. *Gently* move your foot in (Fig. 11.2b) and out (Fig. 11.2c) as far as is comfortable. Return to the starting position and perform this exercise four times.

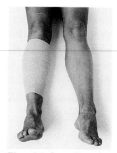

Fig. 11.2a Starting position.

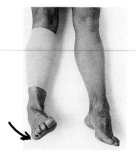

Fig. 11.2b.

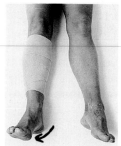

Fig. 11.2c.

RICE

Apply relative rest, ice, compression and elevation following each exercise session. **Have you read the guidelines in chapter five (pages 12, 13 and 14)?**

DAY FOUR

Review your progress

Answer the questions below to review your progress:

- Has your pain become intermittent?
- Do you have less swelling at your injury site?
- Is there increased movement at your ankle?
- Is walking more comfortable?

If you answer **'yes' to all** of the above questions, your shin continues to improve. Progress to DAY FOUR TO DAY EIGHT of the treatment programme. If you answer **'no' to one or more** of the above questions, seek advice from a doctor or physiotherapist.

DAY FOUR TO DAY EIGHT

Start here if your injury is more than three days old

Movement

Gradually increase the exercising of your injured shin. Walk smoothly and with even steps. Perform exercises 11.3 and 11.4 every three hours. When exercising move your injured area to the point of *stretch but not pain*. If you started this treatment programme at DAY ONE, stop exercises 11.1 and 11.2. If you are starting the exercise programme now, follow the guidelines for exercising on page 16.

Exercise 11.3   Position yourself as in Fig. 11.3a and 11.3b with your feet parallel and a shoulder-width apart. Keeping your heels on the ground, slowly bend at your knees and ankles until you feel a *gentle stretch* at your injury site (Fig. 11.3c) and hold for five seconds. Return to the starting position and perform this exercise four times.

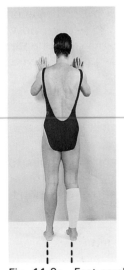

Fig. 11.3a   Feet parallel.

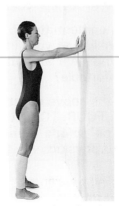

Fig. 11.3b   Starting position.

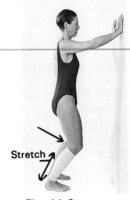

Stretch

Fig. 11.3c.

Exercise 11.4   Position yourself as in Fig. 11.4a with your leg resting on a firm surface. Slowly move your foot in until you feel a *gentle stretch* at your injury site (Fig. 11.4b) and hold for five seconds. Then slowly move your foot out until you feel a *gentle stretch* at your injury site (Fig. 11.4c) and hold for five seconds. Return to the starting position and perform this exercise four times. Keep your leg still to ensure these movements occur only at the ankle.

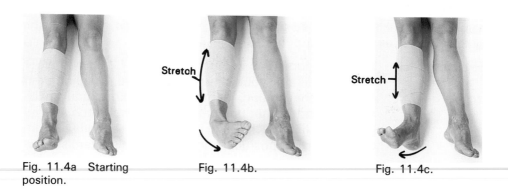

Fig. 11.4a Starting position.

Fig. 11.4b.

Fig. 11.4c.

RICE

Continue with the application of relative rest, ice, compression and elevation following each exercise session. If you are starting the programme now, **refer to DAY ONE — 'RICE' and 'Relative rest' — of this treatment chapter (page 53).** Figs. 11d and 11e demonstrate the application of RICE to your injured shin.

DAY NINE

Review your progress

Answer the questions below to review your progress:

- Do you have intermittent pain only when overstretching your injured area?
- Do you have little or no swelling at your injury site?
- Are you able to perform exercises 11.3 and 11.4 without difficulty?
- Can you walk without limping?

If you answer **'yes' to all** of the above questions, your injury continues to improve. Progress to DAY NINE TO DAY TWENTY-ONE of the treatment programme. If you answer **'no' to one or more** of the above questions, seek advice from a doctor or physiotherapist.

DAY NINE TO DAY TWENTY-ONE

Movement

Return to your daily activities as comfort allows. Do not attempt to run until you can walk briskly without pain or stiffness. Regain and maintain your general fitness by activities that are unlikely to aggravate your injury; for example, swimming or cycling. Stop exercises 11.3 and 11.4. Perform exercises 11.5, 11.6 and 11.7 every three hours. When exercising move your injured ankle to the point of *firm stretch but not pain*, following the guidelines for exercising on page 16.

Exercise 11.5   Position yourself as in Fig. 11.5a and 11.5b with your feet parallel and your injured leg behind. Keeping your heels on the ground, bend your rear knee and ankle. Slowly bend further until you feel a *firm stretch* at your injury site (Fig. 11.5c) and hold for ten seconds. Return to the starting position and perform this exercise four times.

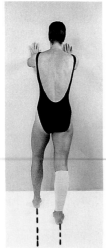

Fig. 11.5a Feet parallel.

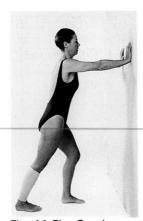

Fig. 11.5b Starting position.

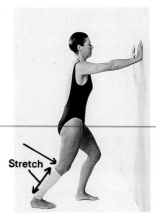

Stretch

Fig. 11.5c.

Exercise 11.6   Position yourself as in Fig. 11.6a and 11.6b with the heel of your injured leg turned out 45 degrees and your injured leg behind. Keeping your heels on the ground, bend your rear knee. Slowly bend your knee further until you feel a *firm stretch* at your injury site (Fig. 11.6c) and hold for ten seconds. Return to the starting position and perform this exercise four times.

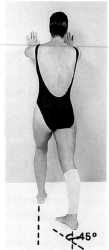

Fig. 11.6a Heels turned out.

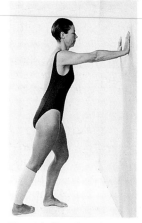

Fig. 11.6b Starting position.

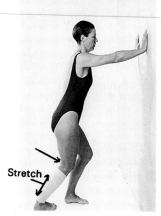

Fig. 11.6c.

Exercise 11.7   Position yourself as in Fig. 11.7a with your injured leg crossed over your other thigh. With your hand slowly point your foot and move it upwards, then apply overpressure until you feel a *firm stretch* at your injury site (Fig. 11.7b) and hold for ten seconds. Return to the starting position and perform this exercise four times.

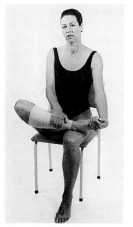

Fig. 11.7a Starting position.

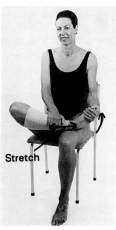

Fig. 11.7b.

RICE

As your pain and swelling decrease, you may reduce the number of times you apply RICE. **Read the guidelines in chapter five (page 14) for when to apply RICE.**

DAY TWENTY-TWO

Review your progress

Answer the questions below to review your progress. Are you able to:

- Perform exercises 11.5, 11.6 and 11.7 with your injured shin almost as well as with your uninjured shin?
- Jog or run without pain?
- Hop without pain?

If you answer **'yes' to all** of the above questions, progress to PREVENTION OF RE-INJURY. If you answer **'no' to one or more** of the above questions, continue with DAY NINE TO DAY TWENTY-ONE of the treatment programme for up to a further three weeks until you answer **'yes' to all** of the above questions. If, after three weeks, you still answer **'no' to one or more** of the above questions, seek advice from a physiotherapist.

PREVENTION OF RE-INJURY

Read chapters 20 and 21 on injury prevention and stretching exercises.

If your work or recreational activities involve running or jumping, a gradual build-up over three weeks is essential. This allows your shin muscle to fully regain the ability to perform these more demanding tasks without the danger of re-injury.

If despite these measures your injury recurs, seek advice from a physiotherapist to determine whether other factors are contributing to this condition.

If you received a direct blow to your shin and intend to return to contact sports, wear shin pads to prevent re-injury.

CHAPTER TWELVE
KNEE INJURIES

The knee is a hinge joint (Fig. 12a) that allows great mobility and relies on strong muscles, firm ligaments and good balance reactions for stability. The main structures that support and guide the knee are:

- Ligaments on either side of the knee (medial and lateral ligaments) and deep inside the knee joint (cruciate ligaments).
- Cartilages (menisci) inside the knee joint.
- The kneecap (patella) in front of the knee joint.
- Muscles, in particular the quadriceps and hamstrings.

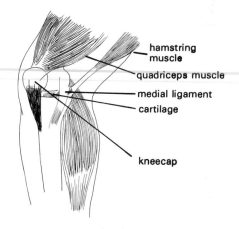

Fig. 12a   Inside view of right knee.

Some knee injuries can be difficult to self-treat. This chapter covers the most straightforward injuries and gives you guidance when to seek medical advice.

The main causes of injury are:

Traumatic injury

A traumatic injury usually involves a twisting or wrenching of the knee joint (Fig. 12b), particularly while you are taking weight through the leg. The medial ligament on the inside of the knee is most commonly sprained,

61

but in more severe injuries the cartilages, cruciate ligaments and the kneecap may also be involved. Other common forms of trauma are kicks or direct blows to the knee which may result in bruising and spraining of the structures surrounding the knee.

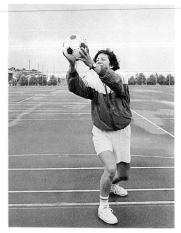

Fig. 12b   Twisting of left knee.

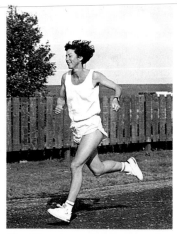

Fig. 12c   Long distance running.

Overuse Injury

An overuse injury of the knee, often referred to as 'runners knee', is usually experienced by teenagers and sports people (Fig. 12c). It starts as a gradual onset of pain behind or around the kneecap and is aggravated by bent-knee activities; for example, jogging, going up and down stairs, sitting or prolonged kneeling. Contributing factors that may lead to overuse injuries are:

    — A sudden increase in work or training activities.
    — An abnormal alignment of the kneecap and the joints in the foot.
    — An imbalance of the muscles that move the knee joint.
    — Worn-out or inappropriate footwear.

> This chapter deals with the self-treatment of straightforward traumatic injuries. Overuse injuries of the knee usually do not respond well to self-treatment alone. If you appear to be suffering from an overuse injury, seek advice from a physiotherapist.

In a typical knee injury you will have experienced the following:

	Traumatic Injury	Overuse Injury
Pain	− At the time of injury a localised sharp pain is felt. This is followed by a constant dull pain. − As the injury heals, the constant pain is replaced by an intermittent pain that is felt only when the soft tissues are over-stretched.	− In teenagers or sports people a dull pain is felt around or under the kneecap when going up or down stairs, during bent-knee activities, during or after sporting activities. − Continued aggravation of the overuse injury leads to a constant dull or throbbing pain.
Swelling and Bruising	Swelling frequently develops around the knee shortly after injury.	A minor swelling may be present.
Movement and Activity	Movements and activities limited by pain are: − Full knee bending. − Full knee straightening. − Squatting.	Usually a full range of movement is present at the knee.

SERIOUS INJURY

Your injury may be serious when:

    a.   You are unable to support any weight through your leg when attempting to walk one hour after the injury occurred.

    b.   Substantial swelling appears *within five minutes* after the injury occurred.

    c.   Your knee gives way or feels unstable during activity.

    d.   Your knee 'locks' and you are unable to fully straighten it.

    e.   Your pain gets worse over two days or you generally feel unwell.

If **one or more** of the above points apply to you, seek medical advice. In the meantime refer to DAY ONE for the application of RICE to limit further damage. If **none of the above points apply to you, you are an ideal candidate for self-treatment.**

SELF-TREATMENT

If this is the first time you are using this book, **read chapters one to seven before commencing self-treatment.** If your injury happened three days ago or less, start the treatment programme at DAY ONE. If your injury happened more than three days ago, start the treatment programme at DAY FOUR TO DAY EIGHT.

DAY ONE

RICE

Apply rest, ice, compression and elevation every three hours. **Read the guidelines in chapter five (pages 12, 13 and 14) for the safe and effective application of ice and cold therapy, compression and RICE.** Figs. 12d and 12e demonstrate the application of RICE to your injured knee.

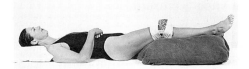

Fig. 12d   Rest, ice and elevation.

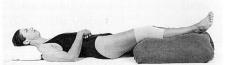

Fig. 12e   Rest, elevation and compression. Start bandaging below knee, finish well above knee.

Relative rest

If walking does not cause any pain, continue to walk with care. If walking is painful, rest for 24 hours. The use of a walking stick (Fig. 12f) will help when you have to walk short distances.

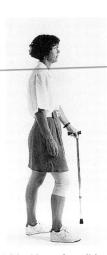

Fig. 12f   Use of walking stick.

DAY TWO

Review your progress

Answer the questions below to review your progress:

- Is your pain intermittent?
- Is your pain constant but less severe than yesterday?
- Are you able to walk short distances with the use of a stick?

If you answer **'yes' to one or more** of the above questions, your knee injury is improving. Progress to DAY TWO TO DAY THREE of the treatment programme. If you answer **'no' to all** of the above questions, seek advice from a doctor or physiotherapist.

DAY TWO TO DAY THREE

Movement

You may begin to exercise your injured knee and walk short distances as comfort allows. Try to walk smoothly and with even steps. When exercising, carefully move your knee. Gentle movement may cause discomfort but should *not produce or increase pain* at your injury site. Perform exercises 12.1 and 12.2 every three hours, following the guidelines for exercising on page 16.

Exercise 12.1   Position yourself as in Fig. 12.1a. *Gently* bend your knee taking your heel towards your buttock as far as is comfortable (Fig. 12.1b). Return to the starting position and perform this exercise four times.

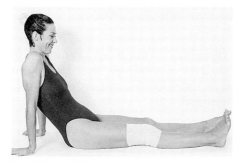

Fig. 12.1a Starting position.

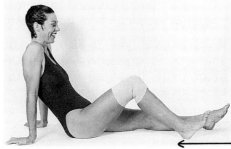

Fig. 12.1b.

Exercise 12.2   Position yourself as in Fig. 12.2a with a rolled towel under
                 your knee. *Gently* lift your foot and straighten your knee
                 as far as is comfortable (Fig. 12.2b). Hold for five
                 seconds. Return to the starting position and perform this
                 exercise four times.

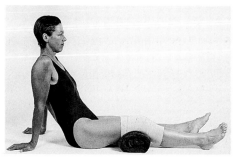
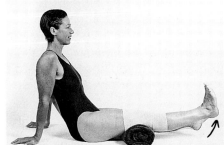

Fig. 12.2a   Starting position.   Fig. 12.2b.

RICE

Apply relative rest, ice, compression and elevation following each exercise
session. **Have you read the guidelines in chapter five (pages 12, 13 and
14)?**

DAY FOUR

Review your progress

Answer the questions below to review your progress:

- Has your pain become intermittent?
- Do you have less swelling at your injury site?
- Is there increased movement at your knee?
- Is walking more comfortable?

If you answer **'yes' to all** of the above questions, your knee continues to
improve. Progress to DAY FOUR TO DAY EIGHT of the treatment
programme. If you answer **'no' to one or more** of the above questions,
seek advice from a doctor or physiotherapist.

DAY FOUR TO DAY EIGHT

Start here if your injury is more than three days old

Movement

Gradually increase the exercising of your injured knee. Walk smoothly and with even steps. Perform exercises 12.3 and 12.4 every three hours. When exercising move your injured area to the point of *stretch but not pain*. If you started this treatment programme at DAY ONE, stop exercises 12.1 and 12.2. If you are starting the treatment programme now, follow the guidelines for exercising on page 16.

Exercise 12.3   Position yourself as in Fig. 12.3a. Bend your knee until you feel a *gentle stretch* at your injury site (Fig. 12.3b) and hold for one second. Return to your starting position and perform this exercise four times.

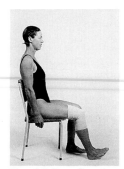 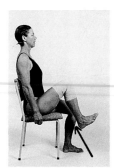

Fig. 12.3a Starting position.   Fig. 12.3b.

Exercise 12.4   Position yourself as in Fig. 12.4a sitting well back in the chair. Slowly lift your foot and straighten your knee until you feel a *gentle stretch* at your injury site (Fig. 12.4b) and hold for ten seconds. Return to the starting position and perform this exercise four times.

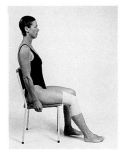 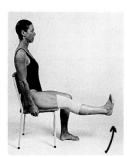

Fig. 12.4a Starting position.   Fig. 12.4b.

RICE

Continue with the application of relative rest, ice, compression and elevation following each exercise session. If you are starting the programme now, refer to DAY ONE—'RICE' and 'Relative rest'—of this treatment chapter (page 64). Figs. 12.d and 12.e demonstrate the application of RICE to your injured knee.

DAY NINE

Review your progress

Answer the questions below to review your progress:

- Do you have intermittent pain only when overstretching your injured area?
- Do you have little or no swelling at your injury site?
- Are you able to perform exercises 12.3 and 12.4 without difficulty?
- Can you walk without limping?

If you answer **'yes' to all** of the above questions, your injury continues to improve. Progress to DAY NINE TO DAY TWENTY-ONE of the treatment programme. If you answer **'no' to one or more** of the above questions, seek advice from a doctor or physiotherapist.

DAY NINE TO DAY TWENTY-ONE

Movement

Return to your daily activities as comfort allows. Do not attempt to run until you can walk briskly, squat and hop several times without pain. Regain and maintain your general fitness by activities that are unlikely to aggravate your injury; for example, cycling or freestyle swimming. If cycling is painful, elevate the seat to allow easier movement at the knee. Stop exercises 12.3 and 12.4. Perform exercises 12.5, 12.6 and 12.7 every three hours. When exercising move your injured knee to the point of *firm stretch but not pain*, following the guidelines for exercising on page 16.

Exercise 12.5   Position yourself as in Fig. 12.5a. Bend your knee, then using your hands slowly pull your heel towards your buttock until you feel a *firm stretch* at your injury site (Fig. 12.5b) and hold for three seconds. Return to the starting position and perform this exercise four times.

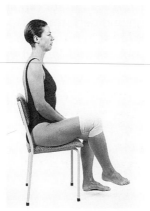
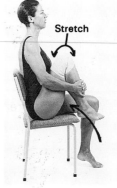

Fig. 12.5a   Starting position.   Fig. 12.5b.

Exercise 12.6   Position yourself as in Fig. 12.6a, sitting well back on a table. Place a light weight (one kilogram or less) around the ankle of your injured leg. A can of beans in a sock or stocking makes an ideal weight. Slowly lift your foot and straighten your knee until you feel a *firm stretch or tension* at your injury site (Fig. 12.6b). Hold for ten seconds. Return to the starting position and perform this exercise four times.

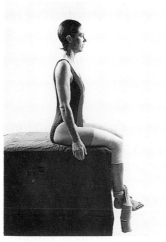
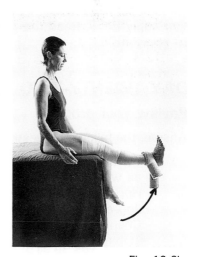

Fig. 12.6a   Starting position.   Fig. 12.6b.

69

Exercise 12.7   Position yourself as in Fig. 12.7a with your feet a shoulder-width apart. Hold onto a table or wall for support. Taking some weight through your injured leg, slowly bend your knees to 45 degrees or until you feel a *firm stretch* at your injury site(Fig. 12.7b). As you do this keep the centre of your knees directly above your second toe (Fig. 12.7c). Hold for ten seconds. Return to the starting position and perform this exercise four times. As your injury improves, you will be able to take more weight through your injured leg when performing this exercise.

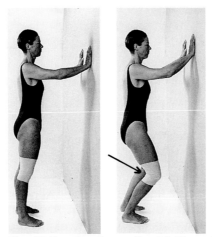 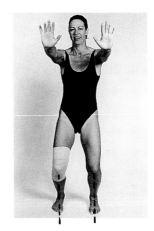

Fig. 12.7a Starting   Fig. 12.7b   Fig. 12.7c Centre of knees
position.   over second toes.

RICE

As your pain and swelling decrease, you may reduce the number of times you apply RICE. **Read the guidelines in chapter five (page 14) for when to apply RICE.**

DAY TWENTY-TWO

Review your progress

Answer the following questions to evaluate your progress. Are you able to:

- Perform exercises 12.5 and 12.6 with your injured knee almost as well as with your uninjured knee?
- Hop and squat without pain?
- Jog and run without pain?
- Change direction suddenly without your knee feeling unstable?

If you answer **'yes' to all** of the above questions, progress to PREVENTION OF RE-INJURY. If you answer **'no' to one or more** of the above questions, continue with DAY NINE TO DAY TWENTY-ONE of the treatment programme for up to a further three weeks until you answer **'yes' to all** of the above questions. If, after three weeks, you still answer **'no' to one or more** of the above questions, seek advice from a physiotherapist.

PREVENTION OF RE-INJURY

Read chapters 20 and 21 on injury prevention and stretching exercises.

If your work or recreational activities involve running or jumping, a gradual build-up over three weeks is essential. This allows your knee to fully regain the ability to perform these more demanding tasks without the danger of re-injury.

Avoid sprinting, jumping and suddenly changing direction when you are not warmed up or feel tired; also avoid squatting or kneeling for long periods as these activities can aggravate your knee.

CHAPTER THIRTEEN

HAMSTRING MUSCLE INJURIES

The hamstrings are a group of three muscles that run down the back of the thigh from the buttock to behind the knee (Fig. 13a). These muscles play an important role in activities involving walking, running or jumping.

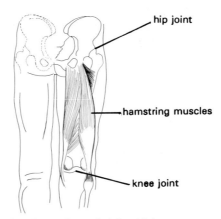

Fig. 13a   Rear view of right thigh.

The main cause of injury is:

Traumatic injury

A traumatic injury involves a strain of the muscle fibres caused by a sudden forceful action, or a bruise caused by a direct blow; for example, a rapid sprint (Fig. 13b) or jump, or a kick to the back of the thigh.

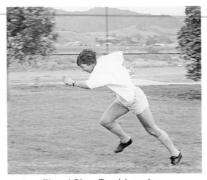

Fig. 13b   Rapid sprint.

In a typical hamstring muscle injury you will have experienced the following:

Traumatic Injury	
Pain	– At the time of injury a localised sharp pain is felt in the back of the thigh. This is followed by a constant dull pain. – As the injury heals, the constant pain is replaced by an intermittent pain that is felt only when the soft tissues are overstretched.
Swelling and Bruising	– Swelling occurs deep in the muscle and often remains undetected. – Bruising may appear a few days after the injury occurs.
Movement and Activity	Movements and activities limited by pain are: – Rapid knee bending. – Toe touching. – Hopping, jumping and sprinting.

SERIOUS INJURY

Your injury may be serious when:

    a.   You feel a tearing sensation at the time of injury and, following this, you are in considerable pain and unable to walk.

    b.   You are unable to support any weight through your injured leg when attempting to walk one hour after the injury occurred.

    c.   You have pain in your lower back or lower leg as well as in the back of your thigh.

    d.   You develop pain, numbness or tingling down your leg or into your foot.

    e.   Your pain gets worse over two days or you generally feel unwell.

If **one or more** of the above points apply to you, seek medical advice. In the meantime refer to DAY ONE for the application of RICE to limit further damage. If **none of the above points apply to you, you are an ideal candidate for self-treatment.**

SELF-TREATMENT

If this is the first time you are using this book, **read chapters one to seven before commencing self-treatment.** If your injury happened three days ago or less, start the treatment programme at DAY ONE. If your injury happened more than three days ago, start the treatment programme at DAY FOUR TO DAY EIGHT.

DAY ONE

RICE

Apply rest, ice, compression and elevation every three hours. **Read the guidelines in chapter five (pages 12, 13 and 14) for the safe and effective application of ice and cold therapy, compression and RICE.** Figs. 13c and 13d demonstrate the application of RICE to your injured hamstring muscle.

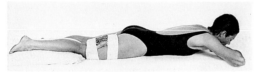

Fig. 13c   Rest and ice.

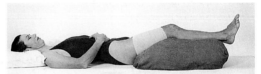

Fig. 13.d   Rest, elevation and compression. Start bandaging just above knee, finish just below hip.

Relative rest

If walking does not cause any pain, continue to walk with care. If walking is painful, rest for 24 hours. The use of a walking stick (Fig. 13e) will help when you have to walk short distances.

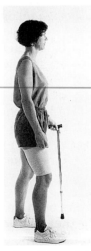

Fig. 13e   Use of walking stick.

DAY TWO

Review your progress

Answer the questions below to review your progress:

  – Is your pain intermittent?
  – Is your pain constant but less severe than yesterday?
  – Are you able to walk short distances with the use of a stick?

If you answer **'yes' to one or more** of the above questions, your hamstring injury is improving. Progress to DAY TWO TO DAY THREE of the treatment programme. If you answer **'no' to all** of the above questions, seek advice from a doctor or physiotherapist.

DAY TWO TO DAY THREE

Movement

You may begin to exercise your injured leg and walk short distances as comfort allows. Try to walk smoothly and with even steps. When exercising, carefully move your leg. Gentle movement may cause discomfort but should *not produce or increase pain* at your injury site. Perform exercise 13.1 every three hours, following the guidelines for exercising on page 16.

Exercise 13.1   Position yourself as in Fig. 13.1a. *Gently* bend your knee taking your heel towards your buttock as far as is comfortable (Fig. 13.1b). Return to the starting position and perform this exercise four times.

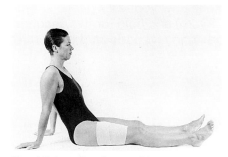

Fig. 13.1a   Starting position

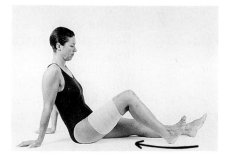

Fig 13.1b

RICE

Apply rest or relative rest, ice, compression and elevation following each exercise session. **Have you read the guidelines in chapter five (pages 12, 13 and 14)?**

DAY FOUR

Review your progress

Answer the questions below to review your progress:

- Has your pain become intermittent?
- Is there increased movement at your hip and knee?
- Is walking more comfortable?

If you answer **'yes' to all** of the above questions, your hamstring muscle injury continues to improve. Progress to DAY FOUR TO DAY EIGHT of the treatment programme. If you answer **'no' to one or more** of the above questions, seek advice from a doctor or physiotherapist.

DAY FOUR TO DAY EIGHT

> **Start here if your injury is more than three days old**

Movement

Gradually increase the exercising of your injured hamstring muscle. Walk smoothly and with even steps. Perform exercises 13.2 and 13.3 every three hours. When exercising move your injured area to the point of *stretch but not pain*. If you started this treatment programme at DAY ONE, stop exercise 13.1. If you are starting the programme now, follow the guidelines for exercising on page 16.

Exercise 13.2   Position yourself as in Fig. 13.2a, clasping your hands under your injured thigh. Keeping your back straight, slowly straighten your knee until you feel a *gentle stretch* at your injury site (Fig. 13.2b) and hold for five seconds. Return to the starting position and perform this exercise four times.

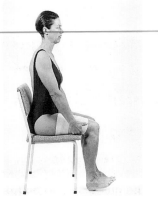

Fig. 13.2a Starting position.

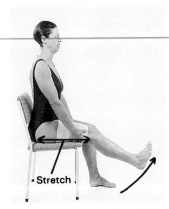

Fig 13.2b.

76

Exercise 13.3   Position yourself as in Fig. 13.3a. Keeping your back straight, slowly lift the heel of your injured leg towards your buttock until you feel a *gentle* stretch at your injury site (Fig. 13.3b) and hold for five seconds. Return to the starting position and perform this exercise four times.

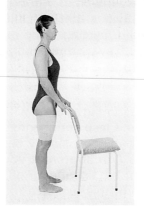
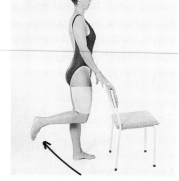

Fig. 13.3a   Starting position   Fig 13.3b.

RICE

Continue with the application of relative rest, ice, compression and elevation following each exercise session. If you are starting the programme now, **refer to DAY ONE—'RICE' and 'Relative rest'—of this treatment chapter (page 74).** Figs. 13c and 13d demonstrate the application of RICE to your injured thigh.

DAY NINE

Review your progress

Answer the questions below to review your progress:

- Do you have intermittent pain only when overstretching your injured area?
- Are you able to perform exercises 13.2 and 13.3 without difficulty?
- Can you walk without limping?

If you answer **'yes' to all** of the above questions, your injury continues to improve. Progress to DAY NINE TO DAY TWENTY-ONE of the treatment programme. If you answer **'no' to one or more** of the above questions, seek advice from a doctor or physiotherapist.

DAY NINE TO DAY TWENTY-ONE

Movement

Return to your daily activities as comfort allows. Do not attempt to run until you can walk briskly and hop several times without pain. Regain and maintain your general fitness by activities that are unlikely to aggravate your injury; for example, swimming or cycling. Stop exercises 13.2 and 13.3. Perform exercises 13.4 and 13.5 every three hours. When exercising move your injured hamstring muscle to the point of *firm stretch but not pain*, follow the guidelines for exercising on page 16.

Exercise 13.4   Position yourself as in Fig. 13.4a with your injured leg on a chair or a table. Clasp your hands behind your back. Keeping your back straight, slowly bend your uninjured leg until you feel a *firm stretch* at your injury site (Fig. 13.4b) and hold for ten seconds. Return to the starting position and perform this exercise four times.

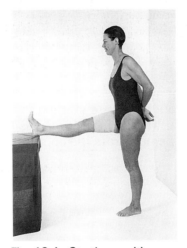
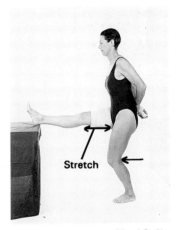
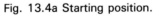

Fig. 13.4a Starting position.   Fig 13.4b.

If Exercise 13.4 does not give a firm stretch at your injury site, refer to page (146) and perform exercise 21.6 but hold for ten seconds.

Exercise 13.5   Position yourself as in Fig. 13.5a with your injured leg
                 on top. Slowly bend your legs using your *uninjured* leg
                 to give firm resistance throughout the movement (Fig.
                 13.5b). Then slowly straighten your legs using your
                 injured leg to give firm resistance throughout the
                 movement (Fig. 13.5c). Perform this exercise four times.

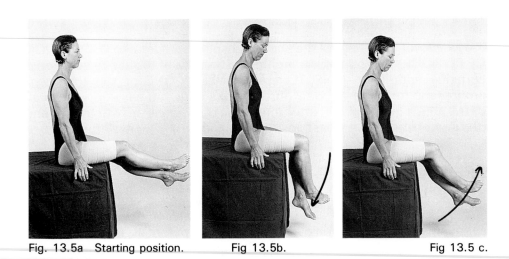

Fig. 13.5a Starting position.   Fig 13.5b.   Fig 13.5 c.

RICE

As your pain and swelling decrease, you may reduce the number of times
you apply RICE. **Read the guidelines in chapter five (page 14) for when
to apply RICE.**

DAY TWENTY-TWO

Review your progress

Answer the following questions to evaluate your progress. Are you able to:

- Perform exercises 13.4 and 13.5 with your injured hamstring muscle almost as well as with your uninjured hamstring?
- Run and sprint without pain?
- Kick a ball without pain?

If you answer **'yes' to all** of the above questions, progress to PREVENTION OF RE-INJURY. If you answer **'no' to one or more** of the above questions, continue with DAY NINE TO DAY TWENTY-ONE of the treatment programme for up to a further three weeks until you answer **'yes' to all** of the above questions. If, after three weeks, you still answer **'no' to one or more** of the above questions, seek advice from a physiotherapist.

PREVENTION OF RE-INJURY

Read chapters 20 and 21 on injury prevention and stretching exercises.

If your work or recreational activities involve running, jumping or sprinting, a gradual build-up over three weeks is essential. This allows your hamstring muscle to fully regain the ability to perform these more demanding tasks without the danger of re-injury.

Avoid sprinting, jumping and suddenly changing direction when you are not warmed up or feel tired.

If despite these measures your injury recurs, seek advice from a physiotherapist to determine whether other factors are contributing to this condition.

CHAPTER FOURTEEN
QUADRICEPS MUSCLE INJURIES

The quadriceps muscle is made up of four large muscles on the front of the thigh that run from the hip to the knee (Fig. 14a). They are a powerful group of muscles that play an essential role in all activities involving walking, running or jumping.

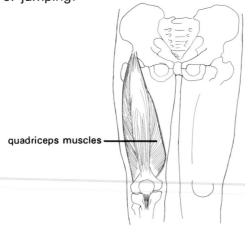

quadriceps muscles ———

Fig. 14a   Front view of right thigh.

The main cause of injury is:

Traumatic injury

A traumatic injury involves a strain of the muscle fibres caused by a sudden forceful action, or a bruise caused by a direct blow; for example, when kicking a ball (Fig. 14b) or receiving a blow to the thigh (Fig. 14c).

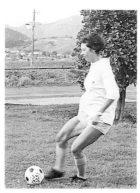

Fig. 14b   Kicking a ball.

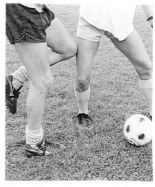

Fig. 14c   Blow to thigh.

In a typical quadriceps muscle injury you will have experienced the following:

Traumatic Injury	
Pain	– At the time of the injury a localised sharp pain is felt on the front of the thigh. This is followed by a constant dull pain. – As the injury heals, the constant pain is replaced by an intermittent pain that is felt only when the soft tissues are overstretched.
Swelling and Bruising	– Swelling occurs deep in the muscle and often remains undetected. – Bruising may appear a few days after the injury occurs.
Movement and Activity	Movements and activities limited by pain are: – Quickly bending or straightening the knee. – Squatting. – Hopping, jumping and sprinting.

SERIOUS INJURY

Your injury may be serious when:

a. You feel a tearing sensation at the time of injury and, following this, you are in considerable pain and unable to walk.

b. There is a marked alteration in the muscle shape after the injury occurred.

c. You are unable to support any weight through your injured leg when attempting to walk one hour after the injury occurred.

d. Your pain gets worse over two days or you generally feel unwell.

If **one or more** of the above points apply to you, seek medical advice. In the meantime refer to DAY ONE for the application of RICE to limit further damage. If **none of the above points apply to you, you are an ideal candidate for self-treatment.**

SELF-TREATMENT

If this is the first time you are using this book, **read chapters one to seven before commencing self-treatment.** If your injury happened three days ago or less, start the treatment programme at DAY ONE. If your injury happened more than three days ago, start the treatment programme at DAY FOUR TO DAY EIGHT.

DAY ONE

RICE

Apply rest, ice, compression and elevation every three hours. **Read the guidelines in chapter five (pages 12, 13 and 14) for the safe and effective application of ice and cold therapy, compression and RICE.** Figs. 14d and 14e demonstrate the application of RICE to your injured quadriceps muscle.

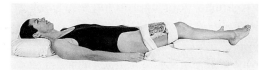

Fig. 14d   Rest, ice and elevation.

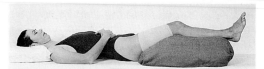

Fig. 14e   Rest, elevation and compression. Start bandaging just above knee, finish just below hip.

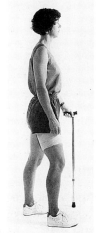

Fig. 14f
Use of walking stick.

Relative rest

If walking does not cause any pain, continue to walk with care. If walking is painful, rest for 24 hours. The use of a walking stick (Fig. 14f) will help when you have to walk short distances.

DAY TWO

Review your progress

Answer the questions below to review your progress:

- Is your pain intermittent?
- Is your pain constant but less severe than yesterday?
- Are you able to walk short distances with the use of a stick?

If you answer **'yes' to one or more** of the above questions, your quadriceps muscle injury is improving. Progress to DAY TWO TO DAY THREE of the treatment programme. If you answer **'no' to all** of the above questions, seek advice from a doctor or physiotherapist.

DAY TWO TO DAY THREE

Movement

You may begin to exercise your injured leg and walk short distances as comfort allows. Try to walk smoothly and with even steps. When exercising, carefully move your leg. Gentle movement may cause discomfort but should *not produce or increase pain* at your injury site. Perform exercise 14.1 every three hours, following the guidelines for exercising on page 16.

Exercise 14.1   Position yourself as in Fig. 14.1a with a rolled towel under your knee. *Gently* straighten your knee as far as is comfortable (Fig. 14.1b) and hold for one second. Return to the starting position and perform this exercise four times.

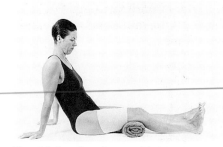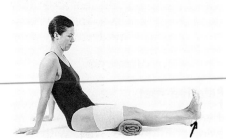

Fig. 14.1a   Starting position.

RICE

Apply relative rest, ice, compression and elevation following each exercise session. **Have you read the guidelines in chapter five (pages 12, 13 and 14)?**

DAY FOUR

Review your progress

Answer the questions below to review your progress:

- Has your pain become intermittent?
- Is there increased movement at your knee?
- Is walking more comfortable?

If you answer **'yes' to all** of the above questions, your quadriceps muscle injury continues to improve. Progress to DAY FOUR TO DAY EIGHT of the treatment programme. If you answer **'no' to one or more** of the above questions, seek advice from a doctor or physiotherapist.

DAY FOUR TO DAY EIGHT

Start here if your injury is more than three days old

Movement

Gradually increase the exercising of your injured quadriceps muscle. Walk smoothly and with even steps. Perform exercises 14.2 and 14.3 every three hours. When exercising move your injured area to the point of *stretch but not pain*. If you started this treatment programme at DAY ONE, stop exercise 14.1. If you are starting this programme now, follow the guidelines for exercising on page 16.

Exercise 14.2   Position yourself as in Fig. 14.2a, sitting well back in the chair. Slowly lift your foot and straighten your knee until you feel a *gentle tension* at your injury site (Fig. 14.2b). Hold for five seconds. Return to the starting position and perform this exercise four times.

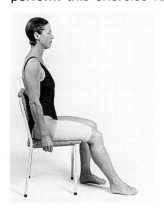 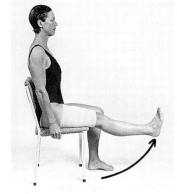

Fig. 14.2a Starting position.

85

Exercise 14.3   Position yourself as in Fig. 14.3a. Keeping your back straight, slowly lift the heel of your injured leg towards your buttock until you feel a *gentle stretch* at your injury site (Fig. 14.3b) and hold for five seconds. Return to the starting position and perform this exercise four times.

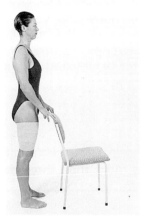 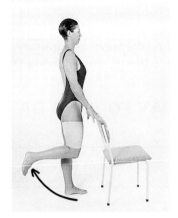

Fig. 14.3a   Starting position.

RICE

Continue with the application of relative rest, ice, compression and elevation following each exercise session. If you are starting the programme now, **refer to DAY ONE—'RICE' and 'Relative rest'—of this treatment chapter (page 83).** Figs. 14.d and 14.e demonstrate the application of RICE to your injured quadriceps muscle.

DAY NINE

Review your progress

Answer the questions below to review your progress:

- Do you have intermittent pain only when overstretching your injured area?
- Are you able to perform exercises 14.2 and 14.3 without difficulty?
- Can you walk without limping?

If you answer **'yes' to all** of the above questions, your injury continues to improve. Progress to DAY NINE TO DAY TWENTY-ONE of the treatment programme. If you answer **'no' to one or more** of the above questions, seek advice from a doctor or physiotherapist.

DAY NINE TO DAY TWENTY-ONE

Movement

Return to your daily activities as comfort allows. Do not attempt to run until you can walk briskly, bend and straighten your knee fully and hop several times without pain. Regain and maintain your general fitness by activities that are unlikely to aggravate your injury; for example, swimming or cycling. If cycling is painful, elevate the seat to allow easier movement at the knee. Stop exercises 14.2 and 14.3. Perform exercises 14.4 and 14.5 every three hours. When exercising move your injured quadriceps muscle to the point of *firm stretch but not pain*, following the guidelines for exercising on page 16.

Exercise 14.4　Position yourself as in Fig. 14.4a with the foot of your injured leg resting on a chair. Hold on to the chair for support with your opposite hand. Keeping your back straight, slowly bend your uninjured knee until you feel a *firm stretch* at your injury site (Fig. 14.4b) and hold for ten seconds. Return to the starting position and perform this exercise four times.

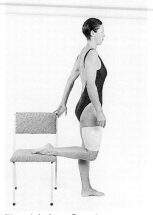 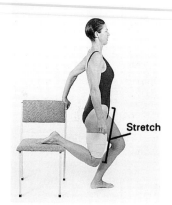

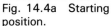

Fig. 14.4a　Starting position.

If you have difficulty with Exercise 14.4 or this exercise does not give a firm stretch to your injury site, refer to page (145) and perform either exercise 21.4 or exercise 21.5 but hold for ten seconds.

Exercise 14.5   Position yourself as in Fig. 14.5a with your feet a shoulder-width apart. Hold onto a table or wall for support. Taking some weight through your injured leg, slowly bend your knees to 45 degrees or until you feel a *firm stretch* at your injury site (Fig. 14.5b). As you do this keep the centre of your knees directly above the second toes (Fig. 14.5c). Hold for ten seconds. Return to the starting position and perform this exercise four times. As your injury improves, you will be able to take more weight through your injured leg when performing this exercise.

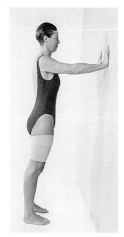

Fig. 14.5a Starting position.

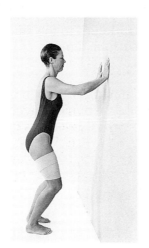

Fig. 14.5c Centre of knees above second toes.

RICE

As your pain and swelling decrease, you may reduce the number of times you apply RICE. **Read the guidelines in chapter five (page 14) for when to apply RICE.**

88

DAY TWENTY-TWO

Review your progress

Answer the following questions to evaluate your progress. Are you able to:

- Perform exercises 14.4 and 14.5 with your injured quadriceps muscle almost as well as with your uninjured quadriceps muscle?
- Go up and down stairs without pain?
- Run and sprint without pain?
- Kick a ball without pain?
- Squat without pain?

If you answer **'yes' to all** of the above questions, progress to PREVENTION OF RE-INJURY. If you answer **'no' to one or more** of the above questions, continue with DAY NINE TO DAY TWENTY-ONE of the treatment programme for up to a further three weeks until you answer **'yes' to all** of the above questions. If, after three weeks, you still answer **'no' to one or more** of the above questions, seek advice from a physiotherapist.

PREVENTION OF RE-INJURY

Read chapters 20 and 21 on injury prevention and stretching exercises.

If your work or recreational activities involve running, jumping or sprinting, a gradual build-up over three weeks is essential. This allows your quadriceps muscle to fully regain the ability to perform these more demanding tasks without the danger of re-injury.

Avoid sprinting, jumping and suddenly changing direction when you have not warmed up or feel tired.

CHAPTER FIFTEEN

GROIN MUSCLE INJURIES

There are a group of muscles that run from the pelvis down to the inside of the thigh. One of these extends as far as the knee (Fig. 15a). These muscles are known as the adductors or groin muscles. They play an important role in controlling the movements of your thigh during running, twisting and jumping activities.

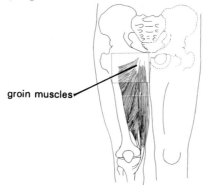

groin muscles

Fig. 15a   Front view of right thigh.

The main cause of injury is:

Traumatic injury

A traumatic injury involves a strain of the muscle or tendon fibres caused by a sudden forceful action; for example, a sudden side-step during sporting activities (Fig. 15b) or slipping on a wet surface (Fig. 15c). Although a groin muscle injury may start as a minor injury, if left untreated it may become a long standing 'nuisance' injury causing discomfort during certain activities; for example, during running, side-stepping, or twisting movements.

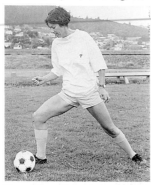

Fig. 15b   Side-step.

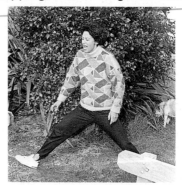

Fig. 15c   Slipping on wet surface.

90

In a typical groin muscle injury you will have experienced the following:

Traumatic Injury	
Pain	— At the time of injury a localised sharp pain is felt at the groin and high on the inside of the thigh. This is followed by a constant dull pain. — As the injury heals, the constant pain is replaced by an intermittent pain that is felt only when the soft tissues are overstretched.
Swelling and Bruising	— Swelling occurs deep in the muscle and often remains undetected. — Bruising may appear a few days after injury.
Movement and Activity	Movements and activities limited by pain are: — Swinging your leg out sideways. — Striding out when walking and running. — Side-stepping when walking and running.

SERIOUS INJURY

Your injury may be serious when:

a   You feel a tearing sensation at the time of injury and, following this, you are in considerable pain and unable to walk.

b.   You are unable to support any weight through your injured leg when attempting to walk one hour after the injury occurred.

c.   Your pain gets worse over two days or you generally feel unwell.

d.   Coughing or sneezing is painful in the groin region.

If **one or more** of the above points apply to you, seek medical advice. In the meantime refer to DAY ONE for the application of RICE to limit further damage. If **none of the above points apply to you, you are an ideal candidate for self-treatment.**

SELF-TREATMENT

If this is the first time you are using this book, **read chapters one to seven before commencing self-treatment.** If your injury happened three days ago or less, start the treatment programme at DAY ONE. If your injury happened more than three days ago, start the treatment programme at DAY FOUR TO DAY EIGHT.

DAY ONE

RICE

Apply rest, ice, compression and elevation every three hours. **Read the guidelines in chapter five (pages 12, 13 and 14) for the safe and effective application of ice and cold therapy, compression and RICE.** Figs. 15d and 15e demonstrate the application of RICE to your injured groin muscle.

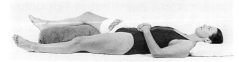

Fig. 15d   Rest, ice and elevation.

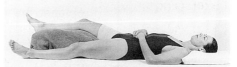

Fig. 15e   Rest, elevation and compression. Start bandaging mid-thigh, finish at groin.

Relative rest

If walking does not cause any pain, continue to walk with care. If walking is painful, rest for 24 hours. The use of a walking stick (Fig. 15f) will help when you have to walk short distances.

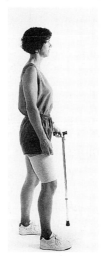

Fig. 15f. Use of walking stick.

DAY TWO

Review your progress

Answer the questions below to review your progress:

- Is your pain intermittent?
- Is your pain constant but less severe than yesterday?
- Are you able to walk short distances with the use of a stick?

If you answer **'yes' to one or more** of the above questions, your groin muscle injury is improving. Progress to DAY TWO TO DAY THREE of the treatment programme. If you answer **'no' to all** of the above questions, seek advice from a doctor or physiotherapist.

DAY TWO TO DAY THREE

Movement

You may begin to exercise your injured leg and walk short distances as comfort allows. Try to walk smoothly and with even steps. When exercising, carefully move your leg. Gentle movement may cause discomfort but should *not produce or increase pain* at your injury site. Perform exercises 15.1 every three hours, following the guidelines for exercising on page 16.

Exercise 15.1   Position yourself as in Fig. 15.1a. Using your hand to support your injured leg, *gently* move your knee out to the side as far as is comfortable (Fig. 15.1b). Return to the starting position and perform this exercise four times.

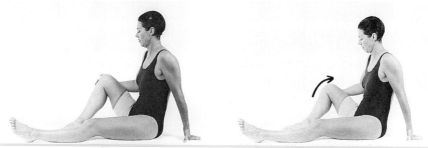

Fig. 15.1a   Starting position.   Fig 15.1b

RICE

Apply rest or relative rest, ice, compression and elevation following each exercise session. **Have you read the guidelines in chapter five (pages 12, 13 and 14)?**

DAY FOUR

Review your progress

Answer the questions below to review your progress:

- Has your pain become intermittent?
- Is there increased movement at your hip?
- Is walking more comfortable?

If you answer **'yes' to all** of the above questions, your groin muscle injury continues to improve. Progress to DAY FOUR TO DAY EIGHT of the treatment programme. If you answer **'no' to one or more** of the above questions, seek advice from a doctor or physiotherapist.

DAY FOUR TO DAY EIGHT

~~Start here if your injury is more than three days old~~

Movement

Gradually increase the exercising of your injured groin muscle. Walk smoothly and with even steps. Perform exercises 15.2 and 15.3 every three hours. When exercising move your injured area to the point of *stretch but not pain*. If you started this treatment programme at DAY ONE, stop exercise 15.1. If you are starting the programme now, follow the guidelines for exercising on page 16.

Exercise 15.2   Position yourself as in Fig. 15.2a. Slowly move your knees towards the ground until you feel a *gentle stretch* at your injury site (Fig. 15.2b) and hold for five seconds. Return to the starting position and perform this exercise four times.

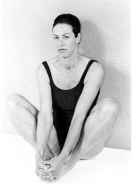

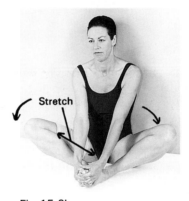

Fig 15.2a Starting position.   Fig 15.2b

Exercise 15.3 Position yourself as in Fig. 15.3a, holding on to a wall for support. Standing on your uninjured leg, slowly move your injured leg out to the side until you feel a *gentle stretch* at your injury site (Fig. 15.3b) and hold for five seconds. Return to the starting position and perform this exercise four times.

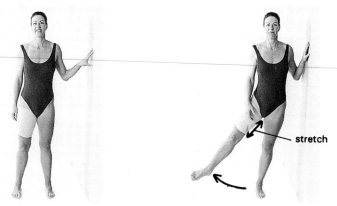

Fig. 15.3a Starting position.   Fig 15.3b

RICE

Continue with the application of relative rest, ice, compression and elevation following each exercise session. If you are starting the programme now, **refer to DAY ONE—'RICE' and 'Relative rest'—of this treatment chapter (page 92)**. Figs. 15d and 15e demonstrate the application of RICE to your injured groin muscle.

DAY NINE

Review your progress

Answer the questions below to review your progress:

- Do you have intermittent pain only when overstretching your injured area?
- Are you able to perform exercises 15.2 and 15.3 without difficulty?
- Can you walk without limping?

If you answer **'yes' to all** of the above questions, your injury continues to improve. Progress to DAY NINE TO DAY TWENTY-ONE of the treatment programme. If you answer **'no' to one or more** of the above questions, seek advice from a doctor or physiotherapist.

DAY NINE TO DAY TWENTY-ONE

Movement

Return to your daily activities as comfort allows. Do not attempt to run until you can walk briskly without pain. Regain and maintain your general fitness by activities that are unlikely to aggravate your injury; for example, freestyle swimming or cycling. Stop exercises 15.2 and 15.3. Perform exercises 15.4, 15.5 and 15.6 every three hours. When exercising move your injured groin muscle to the point of *firm stretch but not pain*, following the guidelines for exercising on page 16.

Exercise 15.4   Position yourself as in Fig. 15.4a. With your forearms slowly push your knees towards the ground until you feel a *firm stretch* at your injury site (Fig. 15.4b) and hold for ten seconds. Return to the starting position and perform this exercise four times.

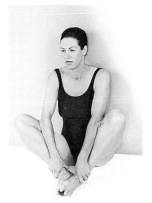

Fig. 15.4a   Starting position.

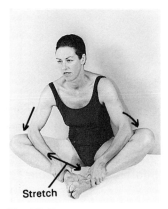

Fig 15.4b

Exercise 15.5   Position yourself as in Fig. 15.5a with your feet parallel and two shoulder-widths apart. Keeping your injured leg straight, move sideways by bending the other leg (Fig. 15.5b). Then slowly lean your body over your straight leg until you feel a *firm stretch* at your injury site (Fig. 15.5c) and hold for ten seconds. Return to the starting position and perform this exercise four times.

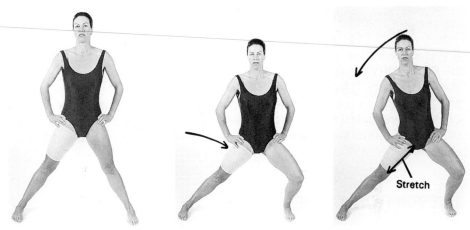

Fig. 15.5a Starting position.   Fig 15.5b   Fig 15.5c

Exercise 15.6   Position yourself as in Fig 15.6a. Squeeze your knees together against your fists until you feel a *firm stretch or tension* at your injury site and hold for ten seconds. Gently ease off and perform this exercise four times.

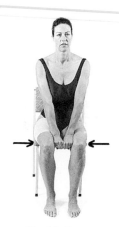

Fig 15.6a

RICE

As your pain and swelling decrease, you may reduce the number of times you apply RICE. **Read the guidelines in chapter five (page 14) for when to apply RICE.**

DAY TWENTY-TWO

Review your progress

Answer the following questions to evaluate your progress. Are you able to:

- Perform exercises 15.4, 15.5 and 15.6 with your injured groin almost as well with your uninjured groin?
- Get in and out of the car without pain?
- Sprint and sidestep without pain?
- Kick a ball without pain?

If you answer **'yes' to all** of the above questions, progress to PREVENTION OF RE-INJURY). If you answer **'no' to one or more** of the above questions, continue with DAY NINE TO DAY TWENTY-ONE of the treatment programme for up to a further three weeks until you answer **'yes' to all** of the above questions. If, after three weeks, you still answer **'no' to one or more** of the above questions, seek advice from a physiotherapist.

PREVENTION OF RE-INJURY

Read chapters 20 and 21 on injury prevention and stretching exercises.

If your work or recreational activities involve running, jumping, side-stepping or sprinting, a gradual build-up over three weeks is essential. This allows your groin muscle to fully regain the ability to perform these more demanding tasks without the danger of re-injury.

Avoid sprinting, jumping and suddenly changing direction when you are not warmed up or feel tired.

If despite these measures your groin injury recurs, seek advice from a physiotherapist to determine whether other factors are contributing to this condition.

CHAPTER SIXTEEN
SHOULDER INJURIES

The shoulder is a ball and socket joint that allows great mobility. This mobility is achieved at the cost of stability. The shoulder has, through the attachments of its muscles, tendons and nerves, a close relationship with the shoulder blade, collar bone and spine (Fig. 16a). For this reason pain felt in the shoulder can arise from the shoulder itself as well as from any of these other structures.

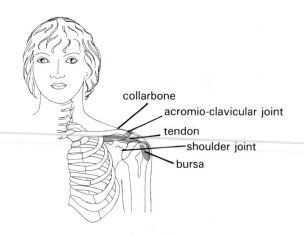

Fig. 16a   Front view of left shoulder.

Some shoulder injuries can be difficult to self-treat. This chapter covers the most straightforward shoulder injuries, and gives you guidance when to seek medical advice.

The two main causes of injury are:

Traumatic Injury

A traumatic injury involves a strain of the tendons around the shoulder joint caused by a sudden forceful action, or bruising from a direct blow to the shoulder; for example, a sudden overstretching of the arm while starting a lawnmower (Fig. 16b) or a fall onto the shoulder joint (Fig. 16c). Such a fall may also affect the joint just above your shoulder, called the acromio-clavicular joint, where the collar bone and the shoulder blade meet.

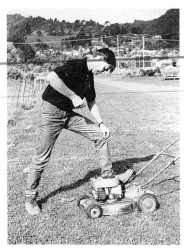

Fig. 16b   Starting a lawnmower.

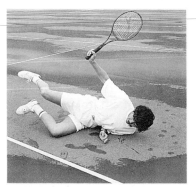

Fig. 16c   Fall onto shoulder.

Overuse Injury

An overuse injury involves an inflammation of the tendons and bursae around the shoulder due to unaccustomed or excessive, repetitive activity; for example, painting a ceiling, pruning a tree (Fig. 16d) or intensive swimming training. Contributing factors which may lead to an overuse injury are:

- A sudden increase or change in training or work activities.
- Prolonged use of the arms above shoulder height.
- Poor neck and shoulder posture.

In the early stages the pain eases with exercise and therefore the problem is often ignored. Continuing the activity results in a long-standing overuse injury. This can take considerable time to heal and may be difficult to self-treat.

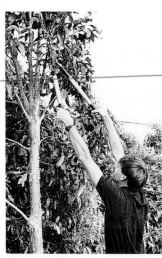

Fig. 16d   Pruning a tree.

In a typical shoulder injury you will have experienced the following:

	Traumatic Injury	Overuse Injury
Pain	– At the time of injury a localised sharp pain is felt. This is followed by a constant dull pain which may spread a few centimeters down the arm. – As the injury heals, the constant pain is replaced by an intermittent pain that is felt only when the soft tissues are over-stretched.	– In the early stages pain is experienced before and after activity but eases during exercise. – Continued overuse leads to a constant dull or throbbing pain, which may spread a few centimeters down from the shoulder.
Swelling and Bruising	– Swelling is usually minor. – Bruising may indicate a serious injury has occurred.	Swelling is rare.
Movement and Activity	Movements and activities limited by pain are: – Raising your arm above your head. – Raising your arm out to the side. – Placing your forearm and hand behind your lower back.	– If the injury is minor, full movement is usually present. – Stiffness may be felt when beginning activity after sleeping or resting. – If the injury is severe, all shoulder movements are limited by pain.

SERIOUS INJURY

Your injury may be serious when:

    a.   Following your injury you are in considerable pain and unable to lift your arm.

    b.   There is an obvious deformity of your injured shoulder.

    c.   You develop pain, numbness or tingling down your arm or into your hand.

    d.   You are unable to lift your arm above shoulder height two days after the onset of the injury.

    e.   Pain prevents you from sleeping or wakes you on successive nights.

    f.   Your pain gets worse over two days or you generally feel unwell.

If **one or more** of the above points apply to you, seek medical advice. In the meantime refer to DAY ONE for the application of RICE to limit further damage. If **none of the above points apply to you, you are an ideal candidate for self-treatment.**

SELF-TREATMENT

If this is the first time you are using this book, **read chapters one to seven before commencing self-treatment.** If your injury happened three days ago or less, start the treatment programme at DAY ONE. If your injury happened more than three days ago, start the treatment programme at DAY FOUR TO DAY EIGHT.

DAY ONE

RICE

Apply rest, ice, compression and elevation every three hours. **Read the guidelines in chapter five (pages 12, 13 and 14) for the safe and effective application of ice and cold therapy, compression and RICE.** Fig. 16e demonstrates the application of RICE to your injured shoulder. Fig. 16f demonstrates a comfortable resting or sleeping position. **If you have a heart condition DO NOT use ice or cold therapy on your shoulders.**

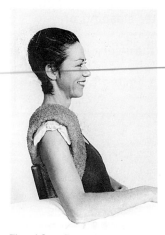

Fig. 16e   Rest, ice and elevation.

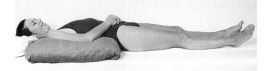

Fig. 16f   Resting position.

Relative rest

Continue to use your arm if this does not cause any pain. If your arm is painful, rest for 24 hours using a sling as support (Fig. 16g).

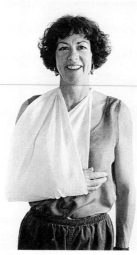

Fig. 16g   Use of sling.

DAY TWO

Review your progress

Answer the questions below to review your progress:

- Is your pain intermittent?
- Is your pain constant but less severe than yesterday?
- Are you able to reach forward with your arm?

If you answer **'yes' to one or more** of the above questions, your shoulder injury is improving. Progress to DAY TWO TO DAY THREE of the treatment programme. If you answer **'no' to all** of the above questions, seek advice from a doctor or physiotherapist.

DAY TWO TO DAY THREE

Movement

You may begin to exercise and use your injured arm for short periods at a time as comfort allows. When exercising, carefully move your arm. Gentle movement may cause discomfort but should *not produce or increase pain* at your injury site. Perform exercise 16.1 every three hours, following the guidelines for exercising on page 16.

Exercise 16.1   Position yourself as in Fig. 16.1a, interlocking the fingers of both hands. *Gently* raise your arms above your head as far as is comfortable (Fig. 16.1b) and hold for one second. Return to the starting position and perform this exercise four times.

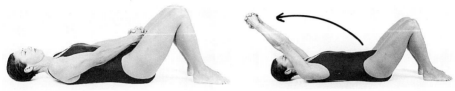

Fig. 16.1a Starting position.   Fig. 16.1b

RICE

Apply relative rest, ice, compression and elevation following each exercise session. **Have you read the guidelines in chapter five (pages 12, 13 and 14)?**

DAY FOUR

Review your progress

Answer the questions below to review your progress:

- – Has your pain become intermittent?
- – Is there increased movement at your shoulder?
- – Is getting dressed more comfortable?

If you answer **'yes' to all** of the above questions, your shoulder injury continues to improve. Progress to DAY FOUR TO DAY EIGHT of the treatment programme. If you answer **'no' to one or more** of the above questions, seek advice from a doctor or physiotherapist.

DAY FOUR TO DAY EIGHT

Start here if your injury is more than three days old

Movement

Gradually increase the exercising of your injured shoulder. Perform exercises 16.2 and 16.3 every three hours. When exercising move your injured area to the point of *stretch but not pain*. If you started this treatment programme at DAY ONE, stop exercise 16.1. If you are starting the programme now, follow the guidelines for exercising on page 16.

Exercise 16.2   Position yourself as in Fig. 16.2a, interlocking the fingers of both hands. Slowly raise your arms above your head until you feel a *gentle stretch* at your injury site (Fig. 16.2b) and hold for one second. Return to the starting position and perform this exercise four times.

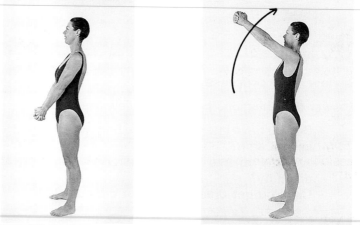

Fig. 16.2a   Starting position.   Fig. 16.2b

Exercise 16.3   Position yourself as in Fig. 16.3a with your injured arm behind your lower back. Slowly move the back of your hand up along your spine until you feel a *gentle stretch* at your injury site (Fig. 16.3b) and hold for one second. Return to the starting position and perform this exercise four times.

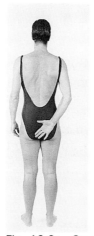
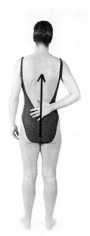

Fig. 16.3a   Starting position.   Fig. 16.3b

RICE

Continue with the application of relative rest, ice, compression and elevation following each exercise session. If you are starting the programme now, refer to **DAY ONE—'RICE' and 'Relative rest'—of this treatment chapter (page 102).** Figs. 16d and 16e demonstrate the application of RICE to your injured shoulder.

DAY NINE

Review your progress

Answer the questions below to review your progress:

- Do you have intermittent pain only when overstretching your injured area?
- Are you able to perform exercises 16.2 and 16.3 without difficulty?
- Can you get dressed without difficulty?

If you answer **'yes' to all** of the above questions, your injury continues to improve. Progress to DAY NINE TO DAY TWENTY-ONE of the treatment programme. If you answer **'no' to one or more** of the above questions, seek advice from a doctor or physiotherapist.

DAY NINE TO DAY TWENTY-ONE

Movement

Return to your daily activities as comfort allows. Avoid prolonged use of your arm above shoulder height. Regain and maintain your fitness by activities that are unlikely to aggravate your injury; for example, cycling, walking or jogging. Stop exercises 16.2 and 16.3. Perform exercises 16.4, 16.5, 16.6 and 16.7 every three hours. When exercising move the injured area to the point of *firm stretch but not pain*, following the guidelines for exercising on page 16.

Exercise 16.4 Position yourself as in Fig. 16.4a with a cloth between the hand of your injured arm and the wall. Slowly slide the hand of your injured arm up the wall until you feel a *firm stretch* at your injury site (Fig. 16.4b) and hold for five seconds. Return to the starting position and perform this exercise four times. As your injury improves, you will be able to progress this exercise by sliding your hand further up the wall and then leaning forward (Fig. 16.4c).

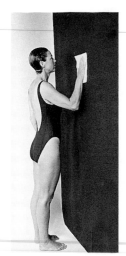
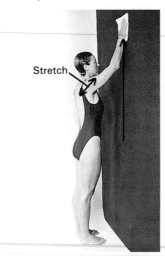
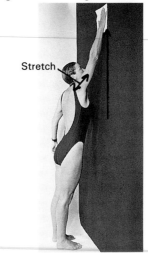

Fig. 16.4a Starting position.

Fig. 16.4b

Fig. 16.4c

Exercise 16.5 Position yourself as in Fig. 16.5a with your injured arm behind your lower back. With your uninjured arm slowly pull your injured arm up until you feel a *firm stretch* at your injury site (Fig. 16.5b) and hold for five seconds. Return to the starting position and perform this exercise four times.

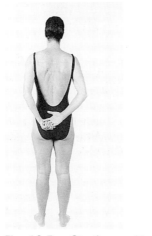
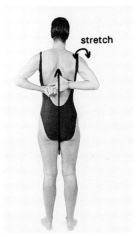

Fig. 16.5a Starting position.

Fig. 16.5b

Exercise 16.6   Position yourself as in Fig. 16.6a. With your uninjured arm slowly pull your injured arm across your chest until you feel a *firm stretch* at your injury site (Fig. 16.6b) and hold for five seconds. Return to the starting position and perform this exercise four times.

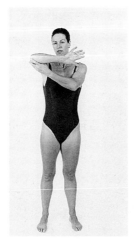

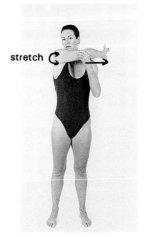

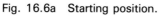

Fig. 16.6a   Starting position.   Fig. 16.6b

Exercise 16.7   Position yourself as in Fig. 16.7a. Push the forearm of your injured arm out against the wall until you feel a *firm stretch or tension* at your injury site and hold for five seconds. Gently ease off and perform this exercise four times.

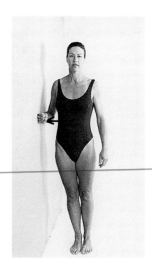

Fig. 16.7a

RICE

As your pain and swelling decrease, you may reduce the number of times you apply RICE. **Read the guidelines in chapter five (page 14) for when to apply RICE.**

DAY TWENTY-TWO

Review your progress

Answer the following questions to evaluate your progress. Are you able to:

- Perform exercises 16.4, 16.5, 16.6 and 16.7 with your injured shoulder almost as well as with your uninjured shoulder?
- Lie on your injured shoulder without pain?

If you answer **'yes' to all** of the above questions, progress to PREVENTION OF RE-INJURY. If you answer **'no' to one or more** of the above questions, continue with DAY NINE TO DAY TWENTY-ONE of the treatment programme for up to a further three weeks until you answer **'yes' to all** of the above questions. If, after three weeks, you still answer **'no' to one or more** of the above questions, seek advice from a physiotherapist.

PREVENTION OF RE-INJURY

Read chapters 20 and 21 on injury prevention and stretching exercises.

If your work or recreational activities involve the use of your arms above shoulder height, a gradual build-up over three weeks is essential. This allows your shoulder to fully regain the ability to perform these overhead tasks without the danger of re-injury.

If you play contact sports, a gradual build-up over three weeks is also necessary. This enables your shoulder to regain the ability to cope with forceful activity.

If you have injured your acromio-clavicular joint, the small joint on the top of your shoulder, strapping may be required for additional support before returning to contact sports. Seek advice on strapping from a physiotherapist.

If despite these measures your shoulder injury recurs, you may have other factors contributing to this condition. Seek advice from a physiotherapist.

CHAPTER SEVENTEEN

ELBOW INJURIES

The elbow consists of three joints that allow bending and straightening of the arm and turning the palm of the hand over and back. The muscles and tendons that work the wrist and fingers attach just above the elbow joint (Fig. 17a).

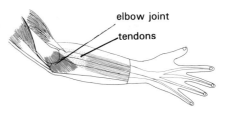

Fig. 17a   View of outer side of right elbow.

The two main causes of injury are:

Traumatic Injury

A traumatic injury usually involves bruising of the elbow from a fall or direct blow, or a sprain of the elbow joint and its surrounding soft tissues; for example, a wrench of the elbow (Fig. 17b) during a contact sport such as karate or judo.

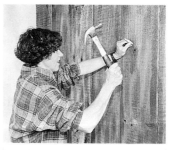

Fig. 17b   Wrench of elbow.

Overuse Injury

An overuse injury is the most common cause of elbow pain and involves inflammation of the tendons and muscles around the elbow due to unaccustomed and excessive, repetitive activity; for example, commencing a racket sport or hammering (Fig. 17c). If the pain is felt on the outer side of the elbow, the condition is commonly called 'tennis elbow'. If the pain occurs on the inner side of the elbow, it is known as 'golfers elbow'.

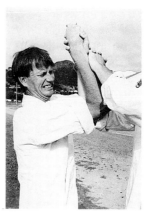

Fig. 17c   Hammering.

110

Contributing factors that may lead to overuse injuries are:
- A sudden increase or change in work or training activities.
- Incorrect technique; for example, a faulty backhand or serving technique when playing tennis.
- A stiff elbow or wrist from a previous injury.

This chapter deals with the self-treatment of straightforward traumatic injuries. Overuse injuries around the elbow do not respond well to self-treatment alone. If you appear to be suffering from an overuse injury, seek advice from a physiotherapist.

In a typical elbow injury you will have experienced the following:

	Traumatic Injury	Overuse Injury
Pain	- At the time of injury a localised sharp pain is felt. This is followed by a constant dull pain. - As the injury heals, the constant pain is replaced by an intermittent pain that is felt only when the soft tissues are overstretched.	- In the early stages pain is experienced when performing gripping or lifting activities. - Continued overuse results in a constant pain which is made worse when attempting to grip or lift.
Swelling and Bruising	- At the time of injury swelling may appear at the injury site. - Bruising may indicate a more serious injury has occurred.	Usually no swelling is present.
Movement and Activity	Movements and activities limited by pain are: - Full bending and straightening of the elbow. - Turning the palm over and back.	Usually full movement at the elbow is present.

SERIOUS INJURY

Your injury may be serious when:

a. Following your injury you are in considerable pain and unable to bear weight through your arm.

b. You develop considerable swelling shortly after the injury occurred.

c. There is an obvious deformity of your injured elbow compared to your uninjured elbow.

d. You feel numbness or tingling in your forearm or hand.

e. Your pain gets worse over two days or you generally feel unwell.

If **one or more** of the above points apply to you, seek medical advice. In the meantime refer to DAY ONE for the application of RICE to limit further damage. If **none of the above points apply to you, you are an ideal candidate for self-treatment.**

SELF-TREATMENT

If this is the first time you are using this book, **read chapters one to seven before commencing self-treatment.** If your injury happened three days ago or less, start the treatment programme at DAY ONE. If your injury happened more than three days ago, start the treatment programme at DAY FOUR TO DAY EIGHT.

DAY ONE

RICE

Apply rest, ice, compression and elevation every three hours. **Read the guidelines in chapter five (pages 12, 13 and 14) for the safe and effective application of ice and cold therapy, compression and RICE.** Figs. 17d and 17e demonstrate the application of RICE to your injured elbow.

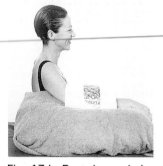

Fig. 17d   Rest, ice and elevation.

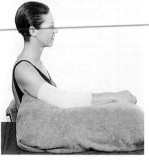

Fig. 17e   Rest, elevation and compression. Start bandaging midway between elbow and wrist, finish midway between elbow and shoulder.

Relative rest

Continue to use your arm if this does not cause any pain. If your arm is painful, rest for 24 hours using a sling as support (Fig. 17f).

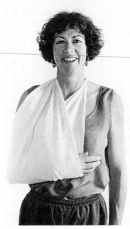

Fig. 17f   Use of sling.

DAY TWO

Review your progress

Answer the questions below to review your progress:

- Is your pain intermittent?
- Is your pain constant but less severe than yesterday?
- Is there increased movement at your elbow?

If you answer **'yes' to one or more** of the above questions, your elbow injury is improving. Progress to DAY TWO TO DAY THREE of the treatment programme. If you answer **'no' to all** of the above questions, seek advice from a doctor or physiotherapist.

DAY TWO TO DAY THREE

Movement

You may begin to exercise and use your injured elbow for short periods at a time as comfort allows. When exercising, carefully move your elbow. Gentle movement may cause discomfort but should *not produce or increase pain* at your injury site. Perform exercises 17.1 and 17.2 every three hours, following the guidelines for exercising on page 16.

Exercise 17.1   Position yourself as in Fig. 17.1a. *Gently* bend (Fig. 17.1b) and straighten (Fig. 17.1c) your injured elbow as far as is comfortable. Return to the starting position and perform this exercise four times.

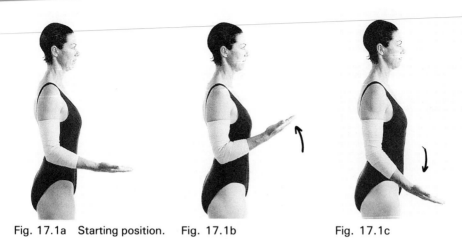

Fig. 17.1a   Starting position.   Fig. 17.1b   Fig. 17.1c

Exercise 17.2   Position yourself as in Fig. 17.2a, holding your injured elbow into your side. *Gently* turn your palm up to the ceiling (Fig. 17.2b) and down to the floor (Fig. 17.2c) as far as is comfortable. Return to the starting position and perform this exercise four times.

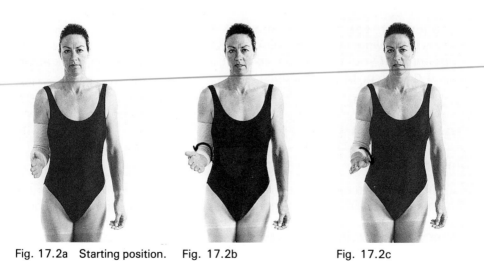

Fig. 17.2a   Starting position.   Fig. 17.2b   Fig. 17.2c

RICE

Apply relative rest, ice, compression and elevation following each exercise session. **Have you read the guidelines in chapter five (pages 12, 13 and 14)?**

DAY FOUR

Review your progress

Answer the questions below to review your progress:

- Has your pain become intermittent?
- Is there increased movement at your elbow?
- Is getting dressed more comfortable?

If you answer **'yes' to all** of the above questions, your elbow continues to improve. Progress to DAY FOUR TO DAY EIGHT of the treatment programme. If you answer **'no' to one or more** of the above questions, seek advice from a doctor or physiotherapist.

DAY FOUR TO DAY EIGHT

> **Start here if your injury is more than three days old**

Movement

Gradually increase the exercising of your injured elbow. Perform exercises 17.3 and 17.4 every three hours. When exercising move your injured area to the point of *stretch but not pain*. If you started this treatment programme at DAY ONE, stop exercises 17.1 and 17.2. If you are starting the programme now, follow the guidelines for exercising on page 16.

Exercise 17.3 Position yourself as in Fig. 17.3a. Slowly bend your injured elbow until you feel a *gentle* stretch at your injury site (Fig. 17.3b) and hold for one second. Then slowly straighten your injured elbow until you feel a *gentle* stretch at your injury site (Fig. 17.3c) and hold for one second. Return to the starting position and perform this exercise four times.

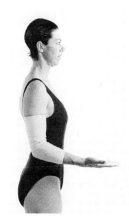 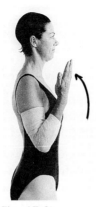 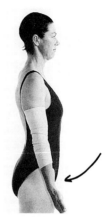

Fig. 17.3a Starting position.   Fig. 17.3b   Fig. 17.3c

Exercise 17.4 Position yourself as in Fig. 17.4a, holding your injured elbow into your side. Slowly turn your palm up to the ceiling until you feel a *gentle* stretch at your injury site (Fig. 17.4b) and hold for one second. Then slowly turn your palm down to the floor until you feel a *gentle* stretch at your injury site (Fig. 17.4c) and hold for one second. Return to the starting position and perform this exercise four times.

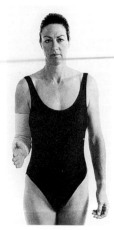 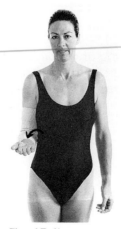 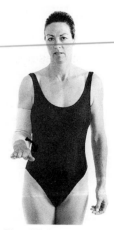

Fig. 17.4a Starting position.   Fig. 17.4b   Fig. 17.4c

RICE

Continue with the application of relative rest, ice, compression and elevation following each exercise session. If you are starting the programme now, **refer to DAY ONE—'RICE' and 'Relative rest'—of this treatment chapter (page 112).** Figs. 17d and 17e demonstrate the application of RICE to your injured elbow.

DAY NINE

Review your progress

Answer the questions below to review your progress:

- Do you have intermittent pain only when overstretching your injured area?
- Are you able to perform exercises 17.3 and 17.4 without difficulty?
- Can you walk normally?

If you answer **'yes' to all** of the above questions, your injury continues to improve. Progress to DAY NINE TO DAY TWENTY-ONE of the treatment programme. If you answer **'no' to one or more** of the above questions, seek advice from a doctor or physiotherapist.

DAY NINE TO DAY TWENTY-ONE

Movement

Return to your daily activities as comfort allows. Avoid strenuous and repetitive activity until you regain normal flexibility, strength and function in your injured elbow. Regain and maintain your fitness by activities that are unlikely to aggravate your injury; for example, using an exercycle, brisk walking or jogging. Stop exercises 17.3 and 17.4. Perform exercises 17.5 and 17.6 every three hours. When exercising move the injured area to the point of *firm stretch but not pain*, following the guidelines for exercising on page 16.

Exercise 17.5 Position yourself as in Fig. 17.5a. Bend your injured elbow as far as you can and slowly apply pressure with the hand of your uninjured arm until you feel a *firm* stretch at your injury site (Fig. 17.5b). Hold for three seconds. Then straighten your injured elbow as far as you can and slowly apply pressure with the hand of your uninjured arm until you feel a *firm* stretch at your injury site (Fig. 17.5c). Hold for three seconds. Return to the starting position and perform this exercise four times.

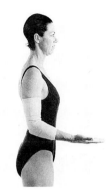 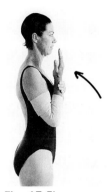 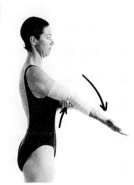

Fig. 17.5a Starting position.   Fig. 17.5b   Fig. 17.5c

Exercise 17.6 Position yourself as in Fig. 17.6a, holding your injured elbow into your side. Turn your palm up to the ceiling as far as you can and slowly apply pressure with the hand of your uninjured arm until you feel a *firm* stretch at your injury site (Fig. 17.6b). Hold for three seconds. Then turn your palm down to the floor as far as you can and slowly apply pressure with the hand of your uninjured arm until you feel a *firm* stretch at your injury site (Fig. 17.6c). Hold for three seconds. Return to the starting position and perform this exercise four times.

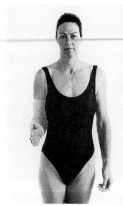 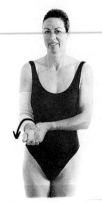 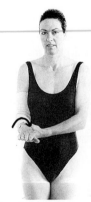

Fig. 17.6a Starting position.   Fig. 17.6b   Fig. 17.6c

118

RICE

As your pain and swelling decrease, you may reduce the number of times you apply RICE. **Read the guidelines in chapter five (page 14) for when to apply RICE.**

DAY TWENTY-TWO

Review your progress

Answer the following questions to evaluate your progress. Are you able to:

- Perform exercises 17.5 and 17.6 with your injured elbow almost as well as with your uninjured elbow?
- Lift and carry a full shopping bag without pain?
- Throw a ball without pain?

If you answer **'yes' to all** of the above questions, progress to PREVENTION OF RE-INJURY. If you answer **'no' to one or more** of the above questions, continue with DAY NINE TO DAY TWENTY-ONE of the treatment programme for up to a further three weeks until you answer **'yes' to all** of the above questions. If, after three weeks, you still answer **'no' to one or more** of the above questions, seek advice from a physiotherapist.

PREVENTION OF RE-INJURY

Read chapters 20 and 21 on injury prevention and stretching exercises.

If your work or recreational activities involve heavy or repetitive lifting, a gradual build-up over three weeks is essential. This allows your elbow to fully regain the ability to perform these more demanding tasks without the danger of re-injury.

If you play contact sports, a gradual build-up over three weeks is also necessary. This enables your elbow to regain the ability to cope with forceful activity.

CHAPTER EIGHTEEN

WRIST INJURIES

The wrist consists of a complex of small bones that allow the hand to move in many directions. The front and back of the wrist are covered by tendons which run from the forearm to the fingers and thumb (Fig. 18a).

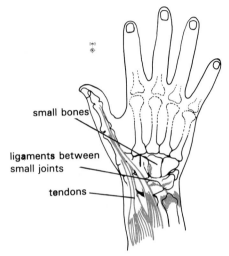

small bones

ligaments between
small joints

tendons

The two main causes of injury are:

Traumatic Injury

A traumatic injury involves bruising of the wrist caused by a direct blow or, more commonly, a sprain of the wrist caused by a fall onto the outstretched hand (Fig. 18b). These injuries usually only affect the soft tissues and small joints of the wrist. However, if you have fallen awkwardly or are in the older age group, some of the bones in the wrist may break with relatively little force.

Fig. 18a   Back view
of right wrist.

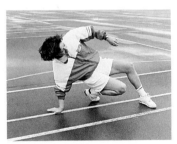

Fig. 18b   Fall onto
outstretched hand.

Overuse Injury

An overuse injury involves an inflammation of the tendons and their covering layers due to unaccustomed or excessive, repetitive activity; for example, starting work on a production line or pruning (Fig. 18c).

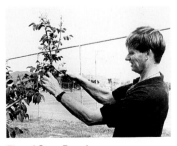

Fig. 18c   Pruning.

Contributing factors that may lead to overuse injury are:

- A sudden increase or change in work or training activities.
- Incorrect technique; for example, when playing a violin.
- Inappropriate equipment; for example, blunt dress making scissors.

In the early stages the pain eases with activity and the problem is often ignored. Continuing the activity results in a long-standing overuse injury. This can take considerable time to heal and may be difficult to self-treat.

In a typical wrist injury you will have experienced the following:

	Traumatic Injury	Overuse Injury
Pain	- At the time of injury a localised sharp pain is felt. This is followed by a constant dull pain. - As the injury heals, the constant pain is replaced by an intermittent pain that is felt only when the soft tissues are overstretched.	- In the early stages a dull pain is experienced before and after activity but eases during exercise. - Continued overuse leads to a constant dull or throbbing pain which is made worse with gripping or lifting activities.
Swelling and Bruising	- At the time of injury there may be a slight swelling of the wrist. - Bruising may indicate a more serious injury has occurred.	Continued overuse may lead to swelling of the lower forearm and wrist.
Movement and Activity	Movements and activities limited by pain are: - Bending the wrist fully backwards and forwards. - Wringing out a wet towel.	- A small loss of movement of the fingers, wrist and thumb may be present. - If more severe, a grating sensation is felt on wrist or thumb movements.

SERIOUS INJURY

Your injury may be serious when:

a. Following your injury you are in considerable pain and unable to grip an object with your hand.
b. You develop considerable bruising or swelling shortly after the injury occurred.
c. There is an obvious deformity of your injured wrist.
d. You feel numbness or tingling in your forearm or hand.
e. You experience considerable pain and weakness in your wrist when attempting to lift a heavy object.
f. Your pain gets worse over two days or you generally feel unwell.

If **one or more** of the above points apply to you, seek medical advice. In the meantime refer to DAY ONE for the application of RICE to limit further damage. If **none of the above points apply to you, you are an ideal candidate for self-treatment.**

SELF-TREATMENT

If this is the first time you are using this book, **read chapters one to seven before commencing self-treatment.** If your injury happened three days ago or less, start the treatment programme at DAY ONE. If your injury happened more than three days ago, start the treatment programme at DAY FOUR TO DAY EIGHT.

DAY ONE

RICE

Apply rest, ice, compression and elevation every three hours. **Read the guidelines in chapter five (pages 12, 13 and 14) for the safe and effective application of ice and cold therapy, compression and RICE.** Figs. 18d and 18e demonstrate the application of RICE to your injured wrist.

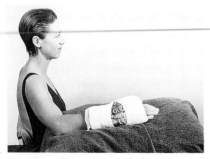

Fig. 18d   Rest, ice and elevation.

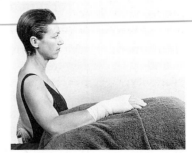

Fig. 18e   Rest, elevation and compression. Start bandaging at base of fingers, finish well above wrist.

Relative rest

Continue to use your wrist and hand if this does not cause any pain. If using your wrist and hand is painful, rest for 24 hours using a sling as support (Fig. 18f).

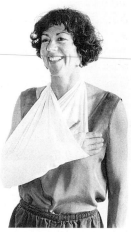

Fig. 18f   Use of sling.

DAY TWO

Review your progress

Answer the questions below to review your progress:
- Is your pain intermittent?
- Is your pain constant but less severe than yesterday?
- Do you have more movement at your wrist?

If you answer **'yes' to one or more** of the above questions, your wrist injury is improving. Progress to DAY TWO TO DAY THREE of the treatment programme. If you answer **'no' to all** of the above questions, seek advice from a doctor or physiotherapist.

DAY TWO TO DAY THREE

Movement

You may begin to exercise and use your injured wrist for short periods at a time as comfort allows. When exercising, carefully move your wrist. Gentle movement may cause discomfort but should *not produce or increase pain* at your injury site. Perform exercises 18.1 and 18.2 every three hours, following the guidelines for exercising on page 16.

123

Exercise 18.1   Position yourself as in Fig. 18.1a. *Gently* move your hand upwards (Fig. 18.1b) and downwards (Fig. 18.1c) as far as is comfortable. Return to the starting position and perform this exercise four times.

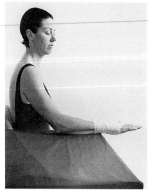
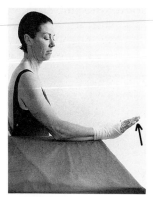
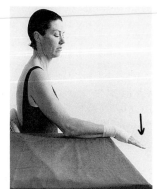

Fig. 18.1a   Starting position.   Fig. 18.1b   Fig. 18.1c

Exercise 18.2   Position yourself as in Fig. 18.2a. Keeping your fingers and thumb together, *gently* move your hand upwards (Fig. 18.2b) and downwards (Fig. 18.2c) as far as is comfortable. Return to the starting position and perform this exercise four times.

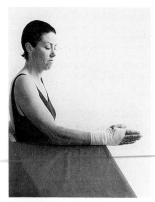
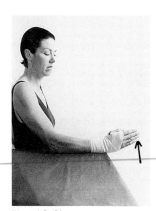
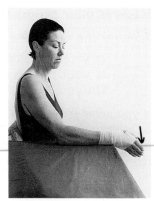

Fig. 18.2a   Starting position.   Fig. 18.2b   Fig. 18.2c

RICE

Apply rest or relative rest, ice, compression and elevation following each exercise session. **Have you read the guidelines in chapter five (pages 12, 13 and 14)?**

DAY FOUR

Review your progress

Answer the questions below to review your progress:

- Has your pain become intermittent?
- Do you have less swelling at your injury site?
- Is there increased movement at your wrist?
- Is lifting light objects more comfortable?

If you answer **'yes' to all** of the above questions, your wrist injury continues to improve. Progress to DAY FOUR TO DAY EIGHT of the treatment programme. If you answer **'no' to one or more** of the above questions, seek advice from a doctor or physiotherapist.

DAY FOUR TO DAY EIGHT

Start here if your injury is more than three days old

Movement

Gradually increase the exercising of your injured wrist. Perform exercises 18.3 and 18.4 every three hours. When exercising move your injured area to the point of *stretch but not pain*. If you started this treatment programme at DAY ONE, stop exercises 18.1 and 18.2. If you are starting the programme now, follow the guidelines for exercising on page 16.

Exercise 18.3   Position yourself as in Fig. 18.3a with your wrist just over the edge of a table and holding on to your forearm. Slowly move your hand upwards until you feel a *gentle* stretch at your injury site (Fig. 18.3b) and hold for one second. Then slowly move your hand downwards until you feel a *gentle* stretch at your injury site (Fig. 18.3c) and hold for one second. Return to the starting position and perform this exercise four times.

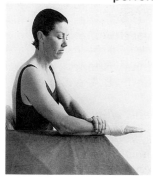 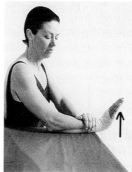 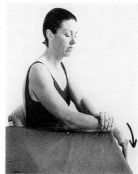

Fig. 18.3a Starting position.   Fig. 18.3b   Fig. 18.3c

Exercise 18.4   Position yourself as in Fig. 18.4a with your wrist just over the edge of a table and holding on to your forearm. Keeping your fingers and thumb together, slowly move your hand upwards until you feel a *gentle* stretch at your injury site (Fig. 18.4b) and hold for one second. Then slowly move your hand downwards until you feel a *gentle* stretch at your injury site (Fig. 18.4c) and hold for one second. Return to the starting position and perform this exercise four times.

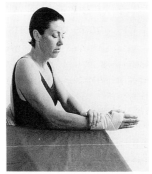 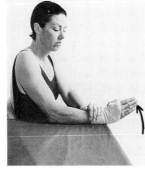 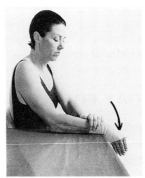

Fig. 18.4a Starting position.   Fig. 18.4b   Fig. 18.4c

RICE

Continue with the application of relative rest, ice, compression and elevation following each exercise session. If you are starting the programme now, **refer to DAY ONE—'RICE' and 'Relative rest'—of this treatment chapter (page 122).** Figs. 18d and 18e demonstrate the application of RICE to your injured wrist.

DAY NINE

Review your progress

Answer the questions below to review your progress:

- Do you have intermittent pain only when overstretching your injured area?
- Do you have little or no swelling at your injury site?
- Are you able to perform exercises 18.3 and 18.4 without difficulty?
- Can you take some weight through your hand without pain?

If you answer **'yes' to all** of the above questions, your injury continues to improve. Progress to DAY NINE TO DAY TWENTY-ONE of the treatment programme. If you answer **'no' to one or more** of the above questions, seek advice from a doctor or physiotherapist.

DAY NINE TO DAY TWENTY-ONE

Movement

Return to your daily activities as comfort allows. Avoid strenuous and repetitive activity until you have regained full flexibility, strength and function in your injured wrist. Regain and maintain your fitness by activities that are unlikely to aggravate your injury; for example, using an exercycle, brisk walking or jogging. Stop exercises 18.3 and 18.4. Perform exercises 18.5, 18.6 and 18.7 every three hours. When exercising move the injured area to the point of *firm stretch but not pain*, following the guidelines for exercising on page 16.

Exercise 18.5   Position yourself as in Fig. 18.5a with the palm of your injured hand on the edge of a flat surface and your other hand on top. Slowly move the elbow of your injured arm up until you feel a *firm* stretch at your injury site (Fig. 18.5b) and hold for three seconds. Then slowly move your elbow down until you feel a *firm* stretch at your injury site (Fig. 18.5c) and hold for three seconds. Return to the starting position and perform this exercise four times.

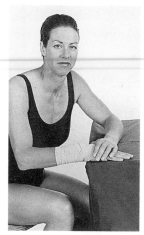

Fig. 18.5a   Starting position

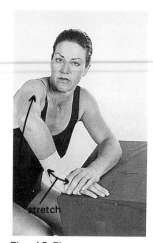

Fig. 18.5b

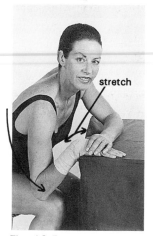

Fig. 18.5c

Exercise 18.6   Position yourself as in Fig. 18.6a with your hand in a fist, thumb tucked in, and holding on to your forearm. Slowly move your fist upwards until you feel a *firm* stretch at your injury site (Fig. 18.6b) and hold for five seconds. Then slowly move your fist downwards until you feel a *firm* stretch at your injury site (Fig. 18.6c) and hold for five seconds. Return to the starting position and perform this exercise four times.

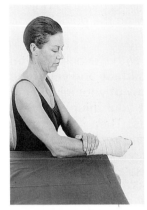

Fig. 18.6a   Starting position.

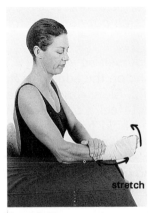

Fig. 18.6b

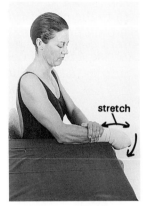

Fig. 18.6c

Exercise 18.7   Take a small towel in both hands. *Firmly* squeeze and rotate the towel in a wringing action (Fig. 18.7a). Rotate the towel with your injured hand four times in one direction, then four times in the opposite direction. Perform this exercise four times.

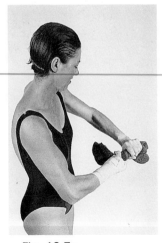

Fig. 18.7a

RICE

As your pain and swelling decrease, you may reduce the number of times you apply RICE. **Read the guidelines in chapter five (page 14) for when to apply RICE.**

DAY TWENTY-TWO

Review your progress

Answer the following questions to evaluate your progress. Are you able to:

- Perform exercises 18.5, 18.6 and 18.7 with your injured wrist almost as well as with your uninjured wrist?
- Take weight through your hand without pain?
- Lift a pot off the stove without pain?

If you answer **'yes' to all** of the above questions, progress to PREVENTION OF RE-INJURY. If you answer **'no' to one or more** of the above questions, continue with DAY NINE TO DAY TWENTY-ONE of the treatment programme for up to a further three weeks until you answer **'yes' to all** of the above questions. If, after three weeks, you still answer **'no' to one or more** of the above questions, seek advice from a physiotherapist.

PREVENTION OF RE-INJURY

Read chapters 20 and 21 on injury prevention and stretching exercises.

If your work or recreational activities involve repetitive or strenuous activity, a gradual build-up over three weeks is essential. This allows your wrist to fully regain the ability to perform these more demanding tasks without the danger of re-injury.

If you play contact sports, a gradual build-up over three weeks is also necessary. This enables your wrist to regain the ability to cope with forceful activity. If you feel your wrist requires additional support, seek advice on strapping from a physiotherapist.

If despite these measures your injury recurs, seek advice from a physiotherapist to determine whether other factors are contributing to this condition.

CHAPTER NINETEEN

FINGER AND THUMB INJURIES

The fingers consist of simple hinge joints. The thumb has greater mobility which makes it more vulnerable to injury (Fig. 19a). Full function of all these joints is necessary for you to perform a great variety of activities from picking up a match to gripping a rope.

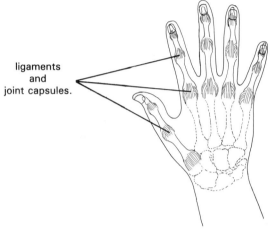

ligaments and joint capsules.

Fig. 19a   Back view of right hand and fingers.

The main cause of injury is:

Traumatic Injury

A traumatic injury usually involves a blow to or overstretching of the fingers or thumb causing a sprain of the ligaments and joint capsule; for example, attempting to catch a ball (Fig. 19b) or falling onto the outstretched fingers or thumb.

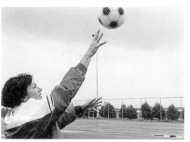

Fig. 19b   Attempting to catch a ball.

In a typical finger or thumb injury you will have experienced the following:

Traumatic Injury	
Pain	— At the time of injury a localised sharp pain is felt. This is followed by a constant dull pain. — As the injury heals, the constant pain is replaced by an intermittent pain that is felt only when the soft tissues are overstretched.
Swelling and Bruising	— Frequently swelling develops around the injured joint shortly after injury. — A few days later bruising may appear around the injured joint.
Movement and Activity	Movements and activities limited by pain are: — Full straightening and bending of the injured finger or thumb.

SERIOUS INJURY

Your injury may be serious when:

    a.   Following your injury you are in considerable pain and unable to grip an object using your injured finger or thumb.

    c.   There is considerable deformity of your injured finger or thumb when compared to your other hand.

    d.   Your pain gets worse over two days or you generally feel unwell.

If **one or more** of the above points apply to you, seek medical advice. In the meantime refer to DAY ONE for the application of RICE to limit further damage. If **none of the above points apply to you, you are an ideal candidate for self-treatment.**

SELF-TREATMENT

If this is the first time you are using this book, **read chapters one to seven before commencing self-treatment.** If your injury happened three days ago or less, start the treatment programme at DAY ONE. If your injury happened more than three days ago, start the treatment programme at DAY FOUR TO DAY EIGHT.

DAY ONE
RICE

Apply rest, ice, compression and elevation every three hours. **Read the guidelines in chapter five (pages 12, 13 and 14) for the safe and effective application of ice and cold therapy, compression and RICE.** Figs. 19c and 19d demonstrate the application of RICE to your injured hand.

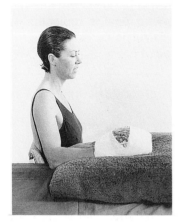

Fig. 19c   Rest, ice and elevation.

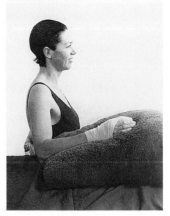

Fig. 19d   Rest, elevation and compression. Start bandaging at tip of injured finger or thumb, finish just above wrist.

Relative rest

Continue to use your hand if this does not cause any pain. If your injured area is painful, rest for 24 hours using a sling as support (Fig. 19e).

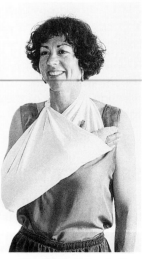

Fig. 19e   Use of sling.

DAY TWO

Review your progress

Answer the questions below to review your progress:

- Is your pain intermittent?
- Is your pain constant but less severe than yesterday?
- Do you have more movement in your finger or thumb?

If you answer **'yes' to one or more** of the above questions, your finger or thumb injury is improving. Progress to DAY TWO TO DAY THREE of the treatment programme. If you answer **'no' to all** of the above questions, seek advice from a doctor or physiotherapist.

DAY TWO TO DAY THREE

Movement

You may begin to exercise and use your injured hand for short periods at a time as comfort allows. When exercising, carefully move your hand. Gentle movement may cause discomfort but should *not produce or increase pain* at your injury site. Depending on the site of your injury perform exercises 19.1 or 19.2 every three hours, following the guidelines for exercising on page 16.

Exercise 19.1 *Finger injuries*	Position yourself as in Fig. 19.1a. *Gently* bend your injured finger down to your palm (Fig. 19.1b) as far as is comfortable, then straighten your injured finger (Fig. 19.1c) as far as is comfortable. Return to the starting position and perform this exercise four times.

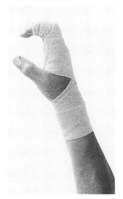
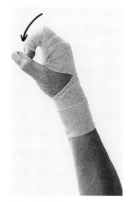
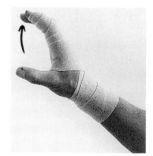

Fig. 19.1a
Starting position.

Fig. 19.1b

Fig. 19.1c

Exercise 19.2	Position yourself as in Fig. 19.2a. *Gently* bend your injured
Thumb	thumb down to your palm (Fig. 19.2b) as far as is
injuries	comfortable, then straighten your injured thumb (Fig.
	19.2c) as far as is comfortable. Return to the starting
	position and perform this exercise four times.

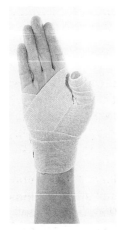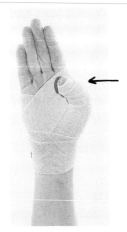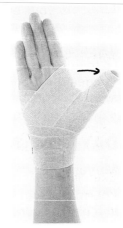

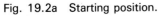

Fig. 19.2a   Starting position.   Fig. 19.2b   Fig. 19.2c

RICE

Apply rest or relative rest, ice, compression and elevation following each exercise session. **Have you read the guidelines in chapter five (pages 12, 13 and 14)?**

DAY FOUR

Review your progress

Answer the questions below to review your progress:

- Has your pain become intermittent?
- Do you have less swelling at your injury site?
- Is there increased movement at your finger or thumb?
- Is grasping light objects more comfortable?

If you answer **'yes' to all** of the above questions, your finger or thumb injury continues to improve. Progress to DAY FOUR TO DAY EIGHT of the treatment programme. If you answer **'no' to one or more** of the above questions, seek advice from a doctor or physiotherapist.

DAY FOUR TO DAY EIGHT

Start here if your injury is more than three days old

Movement

Gradually increase the exercising of your injured finger or thumb. Perform exercises 19.3 or 19.4 every three hours. When exercising move your injured area to the point of *stretch but not pain*. If you started this treatment programme at DAY ONE, stop exercises 19.1 and 19.2. If you are starting the programme now, follow the guidelines for exercising on page 16.

Exercise 19.3
Finger injuries

Position yourself as in Fig. 19.3a. Slowly bend your injured finger until you feel a *gentle* stretch at your injury site (Fig. 19.3b) and hold for one second. Then slowly straighten your injured finger until you feel a *gentle* stretch at your injury site (Fig. 19.3c) and hold for one second. Return to the starting position and perform this exercise four times.

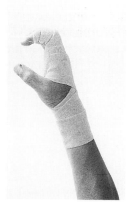

Fig. 19.3a
Starting position.

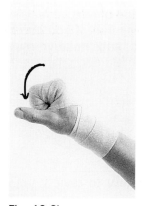

Fig. 19.3b

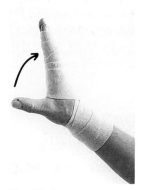

Fig. 19.3c

Exercise 19.4	Position yourself as in Fig. 19.4a. Slowly bend your
Thumb	injured thumb until you feel a *gentle* stretch at your injury
injuries	site (Fig. 19.4b) and hold for one second. Then slowly

straighten your injured thumb until you feel a *gentle* stretch at your injury site (Fig. 19.4c) and hold for one second. Return to the starting position and perform this exercise four times.

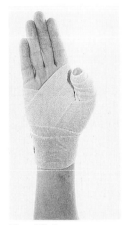
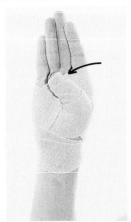
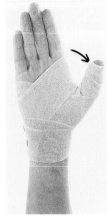

Fig. 19.4a
Starting position.

Fig. 19.4b

Fig. 19.4c

RICE

Continue with the application of relative rest, ice, compression and elevation following each exercise session. If you are starting the programme now, **refer to DAY ONE—'RICE' and 'Relative rest'—of this treatment chapter (page 132).** Figs. 19c and 19d demonstrate the application of RICE to your injured hand.

DAY NINE

Review your progress

Answer the questions below to review your progress:

- Do you have intermittent pain only when overstretching your injured area?
- Do you have little or no swelling at your injury site?
- Are you able to perform exercises 19.3 and 19.4 without difficulty?
- Can you comfortably make a fist?

If you answer **'yes' to all** of the above questions, your injury continues to improve. Progress to DAY NINE TO DAY TWENTY-ONE of the treatment programme. If you answer **'no' to one or more** of the above questions, seek advice from a doctor or physiotherapist.

DAY NINE TO DAY TWENTY-ONE

Movement

Return to your daily activities as comfort allows. Avoid strenuous and repetitive activity until you regain normal flexibility, strength and function in your injured hand. Regain and maintain your fitness by activities that are unlikely to aggravate your injury; for example, using an exercycle, brisk walking or jogging. Stop exercises 19.3 and 19.4. Perform exercises 19.5, 19.6 and 19.7 every three hours. When exercising move the injured area to the point of *firm stretch but not pain*, following the guidelines for exercising on page 16.

Exercise 19.5
Finger injuries

Position yourself as in Fig. 19.5a. Bend your injured finger and slowly apply pressure with your other hand until you feel a *firm* stretch at your injury site (Fig. 19.5b). Hold for three seconds. Then straighten your injured finger and slowly apply pressure with your other hand until you feel a *firm* stretch at your injury site (Fig. 19.5c). Hold for three seconds. Return to the starting position and perform this exercise four times.

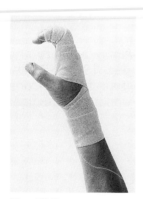

Fig. 19.5a
Starting position.

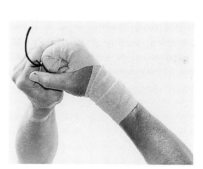

Fig. 19.5b

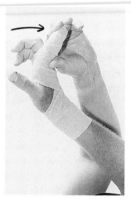

Fig. 19.5c

Exercise 19.6
Thumb
injuries

Position yourself as in Fig. 19.6a. Bend your injured thumb and slowly apply pressure with your other hand until you feel a *firm* stretch at your injury site (Fig. 19.6b). Hold for three seconds. Then straighten your injured thumb and slowly apply pressure with your other hand until you feel a *firm* stretch at your injury site (Fig. 19.6c). Hold for three seconds. Return to the starting position and perform this exercise four times.

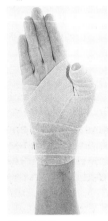

Fig. 19.6a
Starting position.

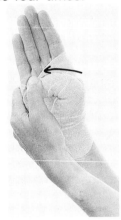

Fig. 19.6b

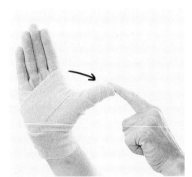

Fig. 19.6c

Exercise 19.7
Finger &
thumb
injuries

Take a small towel in both hands. *Firmly* squeeze and rotate the towel in a wringing action (Fig. 19.7a). Rotate the towel with your injured hand four times in one direction, then four times in the opposite direction. Perform this exercise four times.

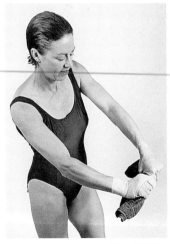

Fig. 19.7a

RICE

As your pain and swelling decrease, you may reduce the number of times you apply RICE. **Read the guidelines in chapter five (page 14) for when to apply RICE.**

DAY TWENTY-TWO

Review your progress

Answer the following questions to evaluate your progress. Are you able to:

- Perform exercises 19.5, 19.6 and 19.7 with your injured hand almost as well as with your uninjured hand?
- Shake hands without pain?
- Lift and carry a full shopping bag without pain?

If you answer **'yes' to all** of the above questions, progress to PREVENTION OF RE-INJURY. If you answer **'no' to one or more** of the above questions, continue with DAY NINE TO DAY TWENTY-ONE of the treatment programme for up to a further three weeks until you answer **'yes' to all** of the above questions. If, after three weeks, you still answer **'no' to one or more** of the above questions, seek advice from a physiotherapist.

PREVENTION OF RE-INJURY

Read chapters 20 and 21 on injury prevention and stretching exercises.

If your work or recreational activities involve repetitive or strenuous activity, a gradual build-up over three weeks is essential. This allows your fingers and thumb to fully regain the ability to perform these more demanding tasks without the danger of re-injury.

If you have injured your fingers or thumb, strapping may be required for additional support before returning to contact sports and sports which involve ball handling. Seek advice regarding strapping from a physiotherapist.

CHAPTER TWENTY

INJURY PREVENTION

The key factors of injury prevention during your work, recreational and sporting activities are:
1. **Fitness for the task.**
2. **Warming up and cooling down.**
3. **Maintaining flexibility.**
4. **Appropriate environment, technique and equipment.**

These four points are particularly important when returning to activity following injury.

Fitness For The Task

If you analyse your daily lifestyle, you will probably find that you spend a considerable amount of time in one position. For example, sitting or standing at work, driving a motor vehicle or watching television at home. These prolonged periods of limited activity result in a loss of general fitness and flexibility. Your body becomes no longer capable of performing strenuous work or recreational activity without risking injury. A programme of regular exercise enables you to maintain the level of fitness and flexibility required to effectively and safely perform more strenuous tasks.

> **Regular exercise provides the necessary link between the sedentary and active aspects of your lifestyle.**

Warming Up And Cooling Down

A warm-up period before beginning heavy or repetitive work, or a recreational activity, prepares your body for the task ahead.

The aim of a warm-up is to limber up and gradually increase your body-temperature to optimal working level. Commence with ten minutes of brisk walking or easy jogging. Follow this by ten minutes of specific stretching exercises. Concentrate on stretching the joints and muscles that you are about to use, in particular those recovered from a recent injury. After completing the stretching exercises, take ten minutes to concentrate on the task ahead and practise the activity, gradually building up to the level of exertion required. Now you are physically and mentally prepared to perform your activity safely and effectively.

Once you have finished your activity, it is equally important to cool down gradually. This allows your body to recover from its recent efforts and reduces the chance of developing soft tissue stiffness and soreness. If your activity has been vigorous, slow down by easy jogging or walking for five minutes. Spend the next ten minutes performing stretching exercises. Emphasise stretching the joints and muscles that have just recovered from injury or feel tight.

> **Thorough warming up and cooling down of a previously injured area plays a vital role in preventing re-injury.**

Maintaining Flexibility

The stretching exercises for warming up and cooling down also maintain your body's general flexibility. Activities such as aerobics, ballet, gymnastics, martial arts and yoga effectively stretch joints and muscles. Most other sporting and recreational activities only work your body through a limited range of movement. An additional programme of stretching exercises is required to maintain full flexibility.

Scar tissue formed following a soft tissue injury has the tendency to shrink and shorten. It is therefore vital that you continue a regular and ongoing stretching programme to maintain normal flexibility, strength and function.

> **Soft tissue injuries that have healed, require regular ongoing stretching to maintain normal flexibility.**

Appropriate Environment, Technique And Equipment

Ensuring that you perform your activities in an appropriate environment with good technique and suitable equipment will minimise the risk of injury.

An appropriate work, home or recreational environment allows you to perform your activities without placing harmful stresses on your body; for example, working at a bench of the correct height will avoid strain on your back, shoulders and arms.

Good technique and appropriate pauses over a period of time enable you to perform your activity efficiently placing minimal stress on your body; for example, using pruning shears close to your body and resting for a few seconds every few minutes when pruning, will place less stress on your shoulders and reduce the chances of developing an overuse injury.

The use of correct equipment will also reduce the chances of injury; for example, wearing appropriate shoes during aerobics or distance running, or protective equipment such as shin pads or gloves during contact sports.

> **A safe and appropriate environment, using the correct technique and equipment, will significantly reduce the chances of injury.**

CHAPTER TWENTY-ONE
STRETCHING EXERCISES

How To Stretch

Effective stretching is performed in a relaxed manner, focussing your attention on the area being stretched. The essential stretching rules are:

Always warm up before stretching.
Do not bounce up and down while stretching.
Perform the stretching exercise to the point of *firm stretch but not pain*.

Commence each stretching exercise slowly. Continue into the movement until you feel a firm stretch. Relax as you hold this position. Then try to stretch a little further until again you feel a firm stretch. Release slowly and rest before repeating.

A series of stretching exercises for warming up and improving your flexibility is illustrated on the following pages. Perform stretching exercises a minimum of three times per week, preferably daily. If you require a more specific programme for your particular activity, seek advice from a physiotherapist.

Stretches For Specific Joints And Muscles

Figure 21.1. Ankle joint stretch

Position yourself as in Fig. 21.1a with your feet apart. Slowly roll on to the outside of your feet until you feel a firm stretch on the outside of your ankles (Fig. 21.1b). Hold for three seconds and perform four times.

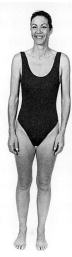

Fig. 21.1a.

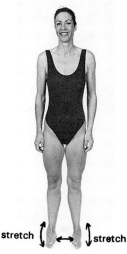

stretch ↕ ↔ ↕ stretch

Fig. 21.1b.

Figure 21.2. Calf muscle stretch—Back of lower leg

Position yourself as in Fig. 21.2a with your feet parallel and the leg to be stretched behind. Keeping your rear knee straight and your heel on the ground, slowly lean forward until you feel a firm stretch along the upper part of the calf of the rear leg (Fig. 21.2b). Hold for 20 seconds and perform four times. Repeat with the other leg.

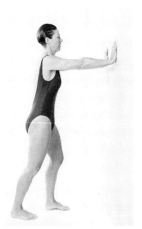

Fig. 21.2a

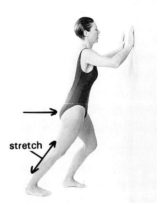

Fig. 21.2b

Figure 21.3. Achilles tendon and calf muscle stretch—Back of heel and lower leg

Position yourself as in Fig. 21.3a with your feet parallel and the leg to be stretched behind. Keeping your rear heel on the ground, slowly bend your rear knee and ankle until you feel a firm stretch along the lower part of the calf of the rear leg (Fig. 21.3b). Hold for 20 seconds and perform four times. Repeat with the other leg.

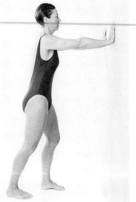

Fig. 21.3a

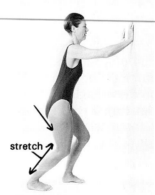

Fig. 21.3b

Figure 21.4. Quadriceps muscle stretch—Front of thigh

Position yourself as in Fig. 21.4a. Taking your weight through your arms, slowly lean back until you feel a firm stretch along the front of the thigh (Fig. 21.4b). You will also feel a stretch along the front of your ankle and foot. Hold for 20 seconds and perform four times.

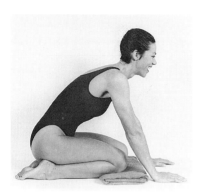

Fig. 21.4a

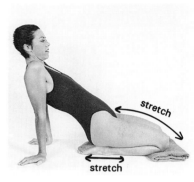

Fig. 21.4b

Figure 21.5. Quadriceps muscle stretch—Front of thigh

Position yourself as in Fig. 21.5a. Keeping your back straight and your knees together, slowly pull your leg behind you until you feel a firm stretch along the front of your thigh (Fig. 21.5b). Hold for 20 seconds and perform four times. Repeat with the other leg.

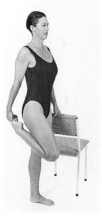

Fig 21.5a

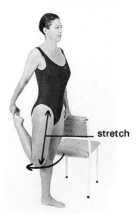

Fig. 21.5b

Figure 21.6. Hamstring muscle stretch—Back of thigh

Position yourself as in Fig. 21.6a, clasping your hands under your thigh and holding your body close to your knee. Maintaining this position, slowly straighten your knee until you feel a firm stretch along the under side of your thigh (Fig. 21.6b). Hold for 20 seconds and perform four times. Repeat with the other leg.

If you have difficulty with this exercise, do exercise 13.2 or 13.4 instead (see pages 76 and 78) but hold for 20 seconds and perform four times.

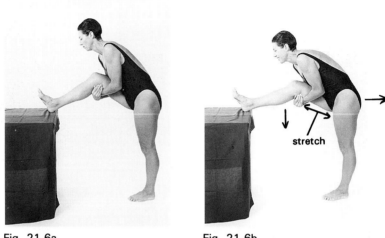

Fig. 21.6a   Fig. 21.6b

Figure 21.7. Groin muscle stretch—Inside of thigh

Position yourself as in Fig. 21.7a. Slowly push your knees toward the ground with your forearms until you feel a firm stretch along the upper inner part of your thighs (Fig. 21.7b). Hold for 20 seconds and perform four times.

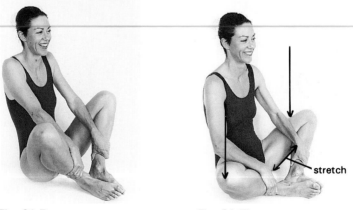

Fig. 21.7a   Fig. 21.7b

Figure 21.8. Groin muscle stretch—Inside of thigh

Position yourself as in Fig. 21.8a with your feet parallel and two shoulder-widths apart. Keeping the leg being stretched straight, move sideways by bending the other leg (Fig. 21.8b). Then slowly lean your body over your straight leg until you feel a firm stretch along the inside of your thigh (Fig. 21.8c). Hold for 20 seconds and perform four times. Repeat with the other leg.

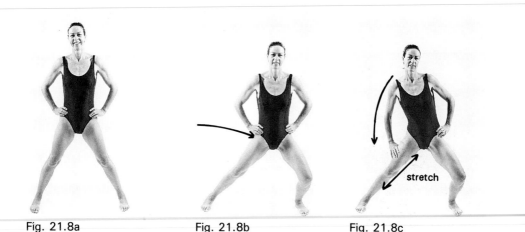

Fig. 21.8a   Fig. 21.8b   Fig. 21.8c

9. Hip flexor muscle stretch—Front of hip

Position yourself as in Fig. 21.9a. You may need to hold on to a solid object for balance. Keeping your back straight, slowly bend your front knee and push your hips forward until you feel a firm stretch at the top of your rear leg (Fig. 21.9b). Hold for 20 seconds and perform four times. Repeat with the other leg.

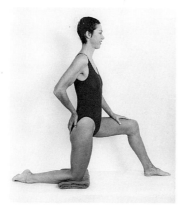
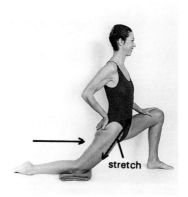

Fig. 21.9a   Fig. 21.9b

147

Figure 21.10. Deep buttock muscle stretch

Position yourself as in Fig. 21.10a, holding onto your knee and ankle. Using even pressure with both hands, slowly pull your knee to your opposite shoulder until you feel a firm stretch on the outside of your hip (Fig. 21.10b). Hold for 20 seconds and perform four times. Repeat with the other leg.

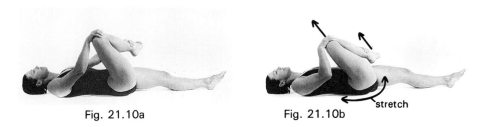

Fig. 21.10a   Fig. 21.10b

Figure 21.11. Outer trunk, hip and thigh stretch

Position yourself as in Fig. 21.11a, placing the leg to be stretched behind the other in a scissor action. Raise the arm of the side to be stretched. You may need a chair for support. Slowly lean over sideways until you feel a firm stretch along the outside of your trunk, hip and thigh (Fig. 21.11b). Hold for 20 seconds and perform four times. Repeat for the other side.

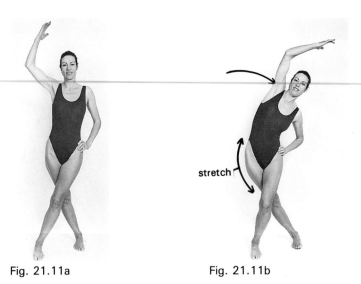

Fig. 21.11a   Fig. 21.11b

Figure 21.12. Low back extension stretch

Position yourself as in Fig. 21.12a, lying flat on your stomach with your hands under your shoulders. Keeping your hips on the ground, slowly push your head, shoulders and upper body up until you feel a firm stretch in your low back (Fig. 21.12b). Hold for one second and perform ten times.

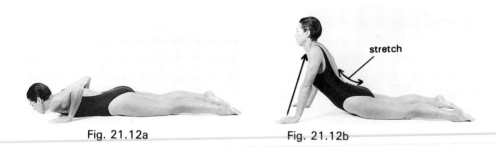

Fig. 21.12a   Fig. 21.12b

Figure 21.13. Low back flexion stretch

Position yourself as in Fig. 21.13a. Slowly pull your knees toward your chest until you feel a firm stretch in your low back (Fig. 21.13b). Hold for one second and perform ten times.

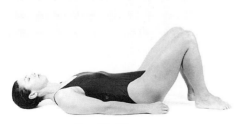
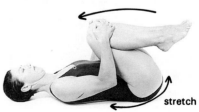

Fig. 21.13a   Fig. 21.13b

Figure 21.14. Inward rotation shoulder stretch

Position yourself as in Fig. 21.14a with the arm to be stretched behind your back. Slowly push this arm up along your back with your other hand until you feel a firm stretch in the shoulder of the arm being pushed up (Fig. 21.14b). Hold for three seconds and perform four times. Repeat with the other arm.

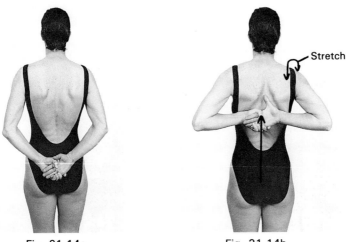

Fig. 21.14a   Fig. 21.14b

Figure 21.15. Horizontal shoulder stretch

Position yourself as in Fig. 21.15a with your thumb pointing to the ground. Slowly pull your arm across your chest until you feel a firm stretch at the back of your shoulder (Fig. 21.15b). Hold for three seconds and perform four times. Repeat with the other arm.

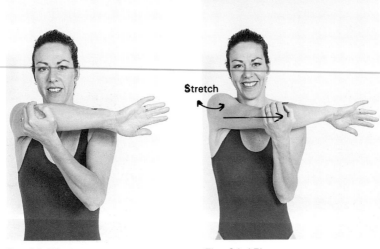

Fig. 21.15a   Fig. 21.15b

Figure 21.16. Vertical shoulder stretch

Position yourself as in Fig. 21.16a. Slowly push your elbow back until you feel a firm stretch under your arm or in your shoulder (Fig. 21.16b). Hold for ten seconds and perform four times. Repeat with the other arm.

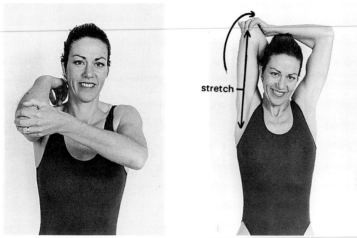

Fig. 21.16a   Fig. 21.16b

Figure 21.17. Forearm and wrist stretch

Position yourself as in Fig. 21.17a, holding one arm straight out in front, palm facing down. Slowly pull the hand and fingers of your straight arm down and back at the wrist until you feel a firm stretch along the upper side of your forearm (Fig. 21.17b). Hold for ten seconds and perform four times. Repeat with the other arm.

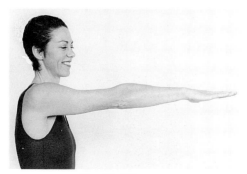
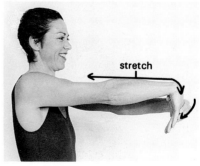

Fig. 21.17a   Fig. 21.17b

Figure 21.18. Forearm and wrist stretch

Position yourself as in Fig. 21.18a, holding one arm straight out in front, palm facing up. Slowly pull the hand and fingers of your straight arm down and back at the wrist until you feel a firm stretch along the upper side of your forearm (Fig. 21.18b). Hold for ten seconds and perform four times. Repeat with the other arm.

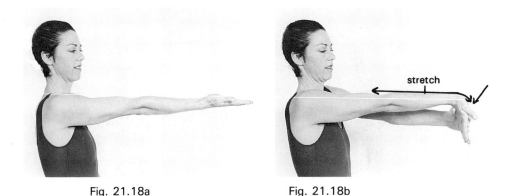

Fig. 21.18a   Fig. 21.18b

Figure 21.19. Neck retraction stretch

Position yourself as in Fig. 21.19a. Move your head backwards, bringing head and neck straight back in line with your trunk (Fig. 21.19b). Slowly push your chin further back with your fingers until you feel a firm stretch in neck and upper back (Fig. 21.19c). Hold for one second and perform ten times.

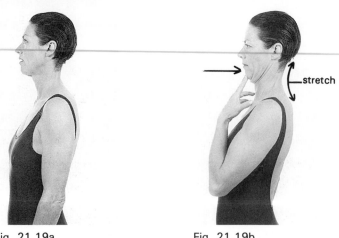

Fig. 21.19a   Fig. 21.19b

Figure 21.20. Neck sidebending stretch

Position yourself as in Fig. 21.20a. Hold on to the seat of the chair with your left hand. With the chin tucked in slowly take your right ear down towards your right shoulder until you feel a gentle stretch on the left side of your neck (Fig. 21.20b). Keep your left shoulder down. Hold for three seconds and perform four times. Repeat for the other side.

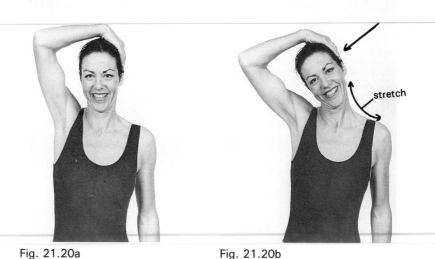

Fig. 21.20a   Fig. 21.20b

Figure 21.21. Neck rotation stretch

Position yourself as in Fig. 21.21a. With the chin tucked in slowly turn towards your left shoulder until you feel a gentle stretch in your neck (Fig. 21.21b). Hold for three seconds and perform four times. Repeat for the other side.

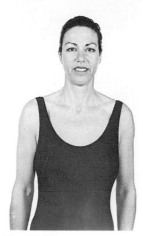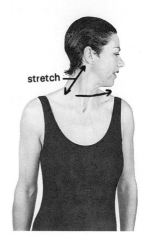

Fig. 21.21a   Fig. 21.21b